Brief Interventions with Bereaved Children

SECOND EDITION

Edited by

Barbara Monroe
Frances Kraus

OXFORD
UNIVERSITY PRESS

D0905720

OXFORD
UNIVERSITY PRESS

Great Clarendon Street, Oxford OX2 6DP

Oxford University Press is a department of the University of Oxford.
It furthers the University's objective of excellence in research, scholarship,
and education by publishing worldwide in

Oxford New York

Athens Auckland Bangkok Bogotá Buenos Aires Cape-Town
Chennai Dar es Salaam Delhi Florence Hong Kong Istanbul Karachi
Kolkata Kuala Lumpur Madrid Melbourne Mexico City Mumbai Nairobi
Paris São Paulo Shanghai Singapore Taipei Tokyo Toronto Warsaw
with associated companies in Berlin Ibadan

Oxford is a registered trade mark of Oxford University Press
in the UK and in certain other countries

Published in the United States
by Oxford University Press Inc., New York

British Library Cataloguing in Publication Data
Data available

Library of Congress Cataloguing in Publication Data
Data available

Typeset in Minion by Cepha Imaging Private Ltd., Bangalore, India
Printed in Great Britain
on acid-free paper by the
MPG Books Group, Bodmin and King's Lynn

ISBN 978–0–19–956164–3

10 9 8 7 6 5 4 3 2 1

Preface

At a conference I attended recently on childhood bereavement, a participant questioned whether, given the contradictory nature of much of the available research data, there was really anything valid we could say about what helps children and their families and carers. This book has been written out of a profound conviction that whilst many questions remain unanswered, there is much that we do know. Children and young people need to have their experiences acknowledged and support to find ways of articulating their story, and to regain some sense of control and confidence in a world that they often experience as chaotic. They need opportunities to remember and where possible a chance to meet others with similar experiences. Support from close friends appears significant. Help needs to be delivered in the context of children's families, existing social relationships and communities, so that these networks are enabled to support over time children whose responses to their loss will change and develop over time.

There is incomplete but developing evidence that the interplay between reactions to grief and other risk factors can lead to negative outcomes for bereaved children, particularly among children who are already vulnerable, both during childhood and later in adult life. The experience of bereavement also seems to have the potential to give some children an increased sense of resourcefulness, maturity, and self-esteem. Research clearly indicates that children's adaptation to bereavement depends much on how their parent or carer manages to support them.

There are inevitable limits to direct service provision and need will always outstrip available specialist resource. The provision of less intensive interventions can make sense as part of a preventive, public health approach. Flexible and accessible short term services delivered at the right time can underpin the strength of bereaved children, young people, and their families, supporting their recovery rather than pathologizing the grief process. Innovative methods of contact will help to extend service reach and respond to individual choice. There is no one-size service that fits all. Every writer in this volume believes that all children and their families and carers have the right to appropriate, culturally sensitive basic information, advice, and support. A few will need much more.

This book resonates with the concept of resilience and the importance of working with the strength and possibilities of children, young people and their families, rather than merely identifying their problems. It is vital that capacity and resource is developed amongst the communities and professional networks in which children already live and in which they can grow and develop, even in the presence of tragic loss. It is also important that bereavement in children and young people is integrated into all aspects of government policy and national service planning.

Society remains afraid of death and adults' fear and silence can leave children's grief invisible and unsupported. We have a responsibility to ensure that bereaved children are not forgotten, their needs left unmet. This underlines the importance of helping parents and families to help their children. Death and loss are part of life. However much we desire to protect children we cannot create for them a world in which these experiences do not exist. Together we can offer children support so that in confronting and learning about death, loss and grief, they develop the emotional capacity and intelligence that will sustain them for the rest of their lives. BM (2004)

Reviewing this preface for the second edition there is little I would wish to alter. Recent practice, research and theorizing, (much of it incorporated into this volume), has tended to confirm the direction of travel already indicated.

In our current uncertain times; faced with global recession, 'natural' disasters like the Australian bushfires and the appalling civilian impact of continued civil war and terrorism in Africa and elsewhere; we need more than ever to treasure and support our children and young people – and their futures. This book has been written in the belief that this activity matters, and that together we can make a difference. BM (2009)

Barbara Monroe
Chief Executive
St Christopher's Hospice and
Director of the Candle Project

Foreword

This book is a remarkable update of *Brief Interventions With Bereaved Children*, edited by Barbara Monroe and Frances Kraus and published in 2005. As Monroe and Kraus report, the field has advanced considerably in the intervening years. The new edition of *Brief Interventions With Bereaved Children* reflects the further development of the overall knowledge and skill base in this area of endeavour and provides an excellent integration of recent advances in evidence and the knowledge base. The theories and approaches described in this book have been well honed by the authors' professional practice with the Candle Project and other child bereavement programmes in Britain. Indeed, most impressive is the number of services that now include a telephone hotline, group education and support, volunteer groups, Internet programmes, brief therapies for individuals and families, and provision of additional services when needed.

Rather than becoming bogged down in a premature discussion of whether mental health interventions focused on current symptoms are effective with bereaved families, the contributing authors ask the more important questions: What services with what intensity are effective? Which services are effective with which individuals? And which ones are effective at which times during the recovery process? Contributors to this volume adopt a quality of life rationale for intervention with bereaved children and families, rather than focusing solely on the reduction of symptoms. They argue that the evidence suggests that these children are clearly stressed and at risk for exacerbation of existing vulnerabilities, and adverse outcomes in both the immediate and longer term. Their broader (or more comprehensive), public health approach is to prevent or mitigate negative consequences and to promote stress-related growth. Components of this approach include timely outreach, focused biopsychosocial assessment, education, supportive and practical intervention, mobilization of networks, community engagement, and follow-up.

Among its many contributions, *Brief Interventions with Bereaved Children* describes three important advances that will guide the field going forward:

- The authors describe how they have learned to meet the particular needs and preferences of their patients and families by combining newer evidence-based approaches with clinical experience.
- They synthesize and analyze the contributions of new theories and research as they apply to bereaved families, and they focus especially on treating

severe reactions, such as posttraumatic stress disorder (PTSD) and complicated forms of grief.

- ◆ They describe how they have implemented a multisystem approach that includes a broad range of interventions, ongoing identification of at-risk populations, and intervention not only at the levels of community, family, and individual child but at the level of national policy as well.

Evidence-based interventions adapted to children's and families' needs and preferences

Rather than apply new interventions in a fashion specified in a manual, the various authors describe a process of listening carefully to what patients and families say they want and need. Outreach is preserved as co-equal in importance to intervention. When the loss is sudden or traumatic, engaging affected children and families is even more difficult. Writers from the Candle Project describe a broad range of outreach methods developed to make services accessible and useful. For example, they have provided child care services on site while parents participated in groups. Instead of the traditional monthly or closed groups, they have conducted three meetings a year for specific populations, such as providers of sibling care. They have developed a large group of trained volunteers who relate their common experiences to families in a creative way that encourages both children and adults to hope that reconstitution of normalcy and good feelings is possible even after the most devastating losses. Others describe sophisticated use of communication via e-mail and the Internet.

Increasing evidence documents that for many reasons, families, especially those confronted with sudden or traumatic loss, are difficult to engage even when they want and need help. For example, existing services may fail to meet a particular family member's needs. Kari and Atle Dyregrov's studies on the impact of a family member's death by suicide found that families clearly said they wanted and needed professionals to be proactive yet flexible and open to the family's specific needs. These families also wanted information about how others had coped with a similar situation, where they could obtain help, and whether assistance was available over longer periods. Our own experience with the widows of fire fighters after the 9/11 World Trade Center disaster also showed that bereaved parents wanted an evaluation of their children's functioning that identified whether the children's behaviours were at a clinical level or were relatively normal reflections of transient stress responses.

Parent guidance interventions that have been evaluated with individuals who have clinical-level symptoms or psychological problems may not be accepted in the same way by individuals in a broad, diverse population, including many whose symptoms are subclinical. The primary aim in the services described is to educate, mitigate distress, and resolve situational and practical problems. In our work with the fire fighters' widows, we found that although principles of parent guidance that have proved to be effective in clinical trials could be used in individual therapeutic conversations, the women often were intolerant of more didactic sessions focused exclusively on parenting. Differences in the acceptability and effectiveness of interventions may depend on the situation and the parent's capacity: e.g., whether the parent is completely overwhelmed and incapable of parenting or is stressed but only wants consultation regarding specific issues. In the current volume, authors offer many examples of the important approach of listening carefully to families' needs and preferences. Feedback was obtained from families and used to modify the interventions' timing, format, frequency, intensity, and content to fit the situations of particular children and families.

Analysis and synthesis of new theory and research on severe reactions

The book provides excellent reviews of new evidence-based approaches that identify what is now known, what is still unknown, and what areas are important for research going forward. For example, the reviews include recently developed concepts involving the impact of trauma and traumatic loss on children in a variety of different situations. Several authors review cognitive behavioural interventions that have shown some effectiveness with traumatized children and they recommend this as an area requiring more research in the future.

William Yule and Patrick Smith discuss newer concepts of PTSD and their application to children: the incidence and prevalence of the disorder, assessment processes, and the concept of traumatic grief when loss is involved. Professionals are cautioned to recognize that interventions found to be effective for PTSD or traumatic loss experienced by adults have not been tested with children. However, those interventions do provide guidance about how traumatic loss experienced by children might be managed in the early period following the loss. The evidence that early intervention prevents later problems is limited. Thus, given the high risk of adverse consequences in these situations, Yule and Smith recommend a programme of planned surveillance and longer-term intervention, rather than a one-time debriefing session.

The prevalence of PTSD in children is low. However, most children experience stress reactions after a traumatic loss. Questions remain concerning whether and, more importantly, how interventions for PTSD might be used for acute stress responses or subclinical conditions. More systematic studies are needed to determine the effectiveness of such interventions in the context of bereaved children. The fact that traumatic stress responses in bereaved children and the efforts to treat them have been recognized represents an important advance in the knowledge base and requires ongoing dissemination and integration of this new information with existing services.

Practitioners will find that the guidelines outlined in the book for managing the reactions of children in the immediate aftermath of a traumatic loss, such as a family member's death by suicide, are especially helpful. The guidelines are informed by evidence, yet are clear and practical. The challenge going forward is to determine when supportive intervention is sufficient to prevent adverse consequences and in what situations a more intensive symptom-focused intervention should be recommended. Are interventions for more severe conditions applicable in modified form for subclinical stress responses? What models are recommended for surveillance in high-risk situations?

Implementing a multisystem and multiple intervention approach

Although the multisystem model is frequently recommended for treatment of bereaved and traumatized children, it is rarely implemented. Services described in this volume clearly demonstrate a multisystem approach to provision of services. Because the model emphasizes a more collaborative or consultative relation to families, it differs from the highly prescriptive multisystem model, which is often recommended for behaviour disorders in children.

The multisystem approach described recognizes that children are dependent and embedded in multiple systems of care and influence. Because it involves intervening at different levels of social organization, the approach optimizes the potential for maximum influence of interventions, thus increasing positive outcomes. The range of services provided in this model also takes into account the many different ways that people cope and increases their ability to find resources and services that are an optimal fit with their culture and family situation. Our own experience with bereaved families of fire fighters after 9/11 is that when multiple services are available, children will use them and find them helpful. Although the frequency of their use was limited, use of the services continued over many years after the traumatic event.

Perhaps one of the most unique and important achievements since the last edition has been the advocacy for bereaved children at the highest levels of governmental policy development in the UK delivered through the collaborative work of the Childhood Bereavement Network. Such a body can disseminate knowledge of bereaved children's needs and experiences to a broad range of professionals, governmental officials, and an informed lay public. Its success suggests this national organizational model could and should be replicated.

Grace Christ, DSW/PhD
Professor
Columbia University School of Social Work

Contents

Contributors

Isobel Bremner
Candle Project Worker,
St Christopher's Hospice,
London, UK

Grace Christ
Professor, Columbia University
School of Social Work,
New York, USA

Gillian Chowns
Visiting Fellow,
Social Work Studies,
University of Southampton, and
Co-director, Palliative Care Works
Farnborough, UK

Atle Dyregrov
Director and Clinical Psychologist,
Center for Crisis Psychology,
Norway

Kari Dyregrov
Researcher and Sociologist,
Center for Crisis Psychology/
Norwegian Institute of
Public Health, Norway

Julie Ellison
Metropolitan Police Detective
Inspector and Candle Project
Volunteer,
London, UK

Frances Kraus
Candle Project Leader,
St Christopher's Hospice,
London, UK

Emma Lupton
Local Authority
Senior Social Worker,
Young Person's Advocate,
Candle Project Advisory Group,
London, UK

Kate MacLeod
National Co-ordinator,
Seasons for Growth,
Scotland, UK

Linda McEnhill
Founder of The National Network
of Palliative Care of People with
Learning Disabilities and Widening
Access Manager,
Help the Hospices,
London, UK

Julia Manning
Candle Project Worker,
St Christopher's Hospice,
London, UK

Barbara Monroe
Chief Executive, St Christopher's
Hospice and Director of the Candle
Project, London, UK; Honorary
Professor, International
Observatory on End of Life Care,
Lancaster University, UK

Rosie Nicol-Harper
Director, SeeSaw (Grief Support
for the Young in Oxfordshire),
Oxford, UK

Alison Penny
Co-ordinator, Childhood
Bereavement Network,
London, UK

Jane Ribbens McCarthy
Reader in Family Studies,
Department of Social Policy and
Criminology, Faculty of Social
Sciences, Open University,
Milton Keynes, UK

Liz Rolls
Senior Research Associate,
Honorary Research Fellow/Chair
Bereavement Research Forum
Department of Natural and Social
Sciences, University of
Gloucestershire,
Cheltenham, UK

Louise Rowling
Honorary Associate Professor,
Faculty of Education and Social
Work, University of Sydney,
Australia

Stewart Sinclair
Social Worker and member of
Candle Project Advisory Group,
London, UK

Patrick Smith
Clinical Psychologist,
Lecturer, King's College London,
Institute of Psychiatry,
London, UK

Peter Speck
Revd Prebendary, Honorary
Senior Lecturer in Palliative Care,
King's College,
London, UK

Julie Stokes
Founder and Clinical Director Lead,
Winston's Wish,
Cheltenham, UK

Di Stubbs
Family Services Team, Winstons
Wish Westmoreland House,
Cheltenham, UK

Patsy Way
Candle Project Worker,
St Christopher's Hospice,
London, UK

William Yule
Emeritus Professor of Applied Child
Psychology, King's College London
Institute of Psychiatry,
London, UK

Chapter 1

Childhood bereavement: the context and need for services

Alison Penny

'This is just a message, to particularly young people in a similar situation as I am, if you've suffered bereavement. This is to say if you are having trouble, don't be afraid to ask for help'.

'Young people need someone to listen to them, and they just need to have clear information'.

(Young people in Childhood Bereavement Network 2002)

The death of a parent, brother, sister, or someone else close is a profound and challenging experience for a young person. Over the last two decades, services to support bereaved children and their families have emerged as a new form of provision (Rolls and Payne 2003). Their growth could be seen simply as an organized, collective expression of the compassion that we feel towards a child who has been bereaved. But why have services developed at this particular point in history? Why do they take the diverse form they do? And why is their coverage still patchy? This chapter will sketch something of the philosophy behind the development of childhood bereavement services, and the specific policy context in England, before looking at current provision.

Setting the scene with prevalence rates is difficult as no national statistics are collected on the number of young people bereaved each year. This lack has been seen as evidence that bereaved children are a hidden or overlooked group (Stokes et al. 1999). Community based samples based on parents' reports of their children's experiences suggest that around 3.5% of those currently aged five to sixteen have been bereaved of a parent or a sibling, and 6.3% have experienced the death of a close friend (Fauth, Thompson and Penny, forthcoming). Childhood bereavement charity Winston's Wish estimates that around

20,000 children under 18 are bereaved of a parent each year (Stokes 2004). Many others have been bereaved of someone else close.

Making the argument for childhood bereavement services

Childhood bereavement services must be able to justify their existence to children and their families, professionals who might refer families to them, and potential funders and supporters. This involves exploring 'implicit assumptions' about the impact of bereavement on children and young people, the value of supporting them through this experience and 'what is considered "best"' for helping them (Rolls and Payne 2004 p31).

Wendy Stainton Rogers outlines three main ways of determining what is in the 'best interests' of a child and thus shaping social policy and provision for children. She identifies these 'discourses of child concern' (p127) as a 'needs discourse', a 'rights discourse', and a 'quality of life discourse'. While childhood bereavement services have often been justified by the 'needs discourse', this has some important limitations, and arguments based on children's rights and quality of life offer helpful supplements.

The 'needs' discourse

A growing body of research has revealed an increasingly complex picture of the impact of bereavement on children and young people, and the range of individual, family, social and structural factors which can affect their experience (Ribbens McCarthy with Jessop 2005). This knowledge has been used to frame children's needs following bereavement (e.g. Worden 1996; Christ 2000; Dyregrov 2008). For example, the Harvard Child Bereavement Study followed 125 parentally bereaved children over a period of two years, matching them to a non-bereaved control group, looking at their responses to the death and exploring the mediating factors affecting the course and outcome of their bereavement. Worden used this to generate a list of needs which 'pertain to most bereaved children' (1996 p140) including adequate information, careful listening, involvement and inclusion and opportunities to remember the person who has died.

As well as describing needs, Worden's list – and others like it – prescribe action, in a move described by Rolls in this volume as a 'move from theory as "insight" to theory as "prescription"'. Empirically based statements of need provide us with a powerful moral obligation to meet those needs, and these can be usefully employed by childhood bereavement services in justifying their interventions.

However, such arguments are rather more precarious than they seem. Statements of need can be deceptively simple (Woodhead 1997) and in practice they often conflict with one another and require careful balancing and flexibility. Such statements imply that if any one need is not met, then a bad outcome will follow, when in fact the complexities and changes in children's lives mean we cannot predict this with any certainty. Too simple a presentation of bereaved children's needs risks criticism from those who argue that such assumptions are unproven (Harrington and Harrison 1999).

Statements of need – while based on the best available evidence at the moment – may be challenged. While they are often presented as universal, statements of need usually reflect cultural assumptions about what is a good outcome for children and young people (Woodhead 1997). Ideas about childhood vary across time and space (Prout and James 1996), and so do ideas about what children need. Even within the same childhood bereavement service, practitioners may hold different 'philosophical positions' on bereavement and on children (Rolls and Payne 2004 p311). In their everyday lives, bereaved children may have to negotiate several different adult views about their needs, or adult views that conflict with their own understanding of their needs.

> My mum helped me because she was always open to talk about when it happened and when my dad was ill she told us everything that happened. Some of my mum's friends said she was too open with us and she shouldn't tell us as much.
>
> (Young person in Childhood Bereavement Network 2003)

Current debates around the role of expressing emotions in dealing with bereavement have implications for interventions (Sandler et al. 2008).

Statements of need do not necessarily justify an organized service response: a wide range of people around an individual child have the potential to be involved in meeting their needs, including family, friends, and the school community. Indeed Worden does not support the provision of specialist services to all children: given that only one third of the children in his study fell into the 'at-risk' group with high levels of emotional or behavioural difficulties at any time during the first two years of their bereavement, he concludes that 'not only is this first approach not needed, it is not cost effective' (p150).

He discusses two alternative approaches to providing services. One is to wait until a child is showing difficulties and then to offer intervention. This requires children to be showing 'an observable level of emotional/behavioural distress before intervention is offered' (p151) which makes the targeting less acceptable. Stokes also points out (2004) that this approach suggests that certain behaviours warrant intervention while others do not, which could result in some children missing out on services that could benefit them.

Worden's preferred model is to use a screening instrument to identify the children most at risk and to offer preventative intervention to them. Again, Stokes points out difficulties with this approach, including concerns about the validity and reliability of a screening tool that must capture an accurate picture of a family's needs but is used at a particular point in time. She concludes 'would the family measured to be 'coping just fine' not be offered any support? If so, this may not necessarily be a view that accurately reflects the experience of the family' (2004 p37).

There are clearly difficulties in using a 'needs discourse' alone to justify services for bereaved children and young people when resources are scarce.

The 'rights' discourse

Rights-based arguments offer an alternative way of justifying services. In particular, this approach views children not as 'a bundle of "needs" that must be met' (Stainton Rogers 2004 p134) but as citizens and social actors capable of holding views and making decisions about their own lives, entitled to rights and respect.

Children's rights are enshrined in the UN Convention of the Rights of the Child (1989) which upholds their rights to the provision of services to promote their healthy development, protection from abuse and exploitation, and participation in decisions about matters affecting their lives (Stainton Rogers 2004 p135).

The Childhood Bereavement Network is the national co-ordinating body for those working with bereaved children in the UK. Its Belief Statement justifies childhood bereavement services in this way as part of a suite of support.

However, this Statement exposes one of the criticisms made of arguments based on moral rights, that without a legal framework to identify who is responsible for meeting those rights, such statements can be no more than aspirations (Axford 2008).

A further complication is that children's rights sometimes conflict with one another and – like their needs – require careful balancing. For example, a child's right to be protected from a situation which adults consider to be potentially harmful could be in conflict with her right to be involved and included. The provision of services may still be based on adults' views about what children need, and we have already seen how these can differ. How is a bereaved young person's right to receive a potentially beneficial service balanced against his right to choose whether to participate?

> After the first session I just didn't want to come back, but I stuck with it and I did come back and I'm really grateful now.

> (Young person in Childhood Bereavement Network 2002)

Box 1.1 CBN belief statement

We believe that all children have the right to information, guidance and support to enable them to manage the impact of death on their lives

Further, in line with the principles of the UN Convention on the Rights of the Child 1989, the Children Act 1989, the Children (Northern Ireland) Order 1995 and the Children (Scotland) Act 1995 we believe any information, guidance and support offered to children should

- ◆ acknowledge the child's grief and experience of loss as a result of death
- ◆ be responsive to the child's needs, views and opinions
- ◆ respect the child's family and immediate social situation, and their culture, language, beliefs and religious background
- ◆ seek to promote self esteem and self confidence, and develop communication, decision making and other life skills
- ◆ be viewed as part of a continuous learning experienced for the child, contributing to the development of the child's knowledge and understanding as they grow into adulthood
- ◆ aim, wherever possible, appropriate and feasible, to involve family members, other caregivers and any professionals working with the individual child in a wider social context.

If this information, guidance, and support is offered as a service by an organisation or in a professional context, it should be

- ◆ provided by people who have had appropriate training and who are adequately supported
- ◆ provided in an appropriately supportive, safe and non-discriminatory context
- ◆ regularly monitored, evaluated and reviewed.

Other dilemmas faced by practitioners in upholding children's rights are where these seem to be in conflict with their parents' (see Chowns 2009 in this volume). A child's right to be informed about her mother's imminent death could conflict with her parent's right to confidentiality about her condition.

The 'quality of life' discourse

Stainton Rogers suggests the 'quality of life' discourse is more promising in making decisions about the best interests of a child, as it resolves some of the conflicts inherent in 'needs' and 'rights' based approaches. This discourse is used particularly in healthcare settings to inform decisions about apportioning resources in the treatment of chronic conditions and palliative care, where improving the quality of the patient's life is the object rather than seeking to cure.

She argues that such an approach accommodates differing value systems, avoiding the universalizing tendencies of the previous discourses and acknowledging that children's welfare is always contextual: it 'cannot be fostered in isolation, but has to take into account the concerns, values, resources and limitations of the families and communities in which children are reared and cared for' (p137). This holistic approach links to ideas about promoting resilience – helping children to overcome adversity and thrive whatever life throws at them – which are particularly relevant when thinking about bereaved children (Stokes 2007). It allows interventions to be framed positively, building on bereaved children and families' strengths and acknowledging their potential for growth and development. Justifying services in terms of children's needs alone can risk pathologizing bereavement, and the quality of life discourse offers an appealing supplement by asking not 'how can we minimize the risks to this child?' but 'how can we improve the quality of this child's life?'

Currier et al.'s meta-analysis of controlled outcome research on childhood bereavement interventions concluded that those not targeted at ' "high risk" children or children already showing signs of difficulty' (2007 p257) did not have significant effects. However, they pointed out that the outcome measures used by the participating studies were 'focused almost exclusively on outcomes defined in terms of psychiatric symptoms or general behavioural disorders' (p258) and wondered whether the researchers would have noted more changes if they had used other measures tailored to the bereavement experience. Stainton Rogers argues that using the quality of life discourse involves careful listening to children and families about their views and experiences of services, which should be judged against their own hopes and expectations as well as those of the professionals devising or providing support. There is an urgent need to develop outcome measures for services which can capture this (Rolls 2007b), building on children and parents' evaluations which reveal the myriad – sometimes unexpected – ways in which interventions make a difference to their lives, over long periods of time (Sandler et al. 2008, Rolls and Payne 2007).

> After the death of my auntie…I felt in myself that I became angry very easily but going through counselling helped me control my anger…Six months ago I wouldn't have thought that I would be able to listen to my auntie's songs that were played at her funeral without feeling sad, but I can.
>
> (Young person in Childhood Bereavement Network 2004)

> We spent the weekend with everybody who's in the same situation as us and we could let out our feelings and everything and say what we thought without anybody teasing us about whether your mum or dad had died.
>
> (Young person in Childhood Bereavement Network 2003)

Improving children and families' quality of life justifies making services available to all bereaved children, provided they are sufficiently flexible to take into account different and changing circumstances, and work in partnership with families, schools, communities, and children themselves. It also justifies some targeting of resources to those children and young people facing particular disadvantage (Ribbens McCarthy with Jessop 2005).

The policy context

National and local policy provides a context to the philosophical debates outlined above. In England, the government's Every Child Matters change programme (www.everychildmatters.gov.uk) has reformed the organization and delivery of children's services across statutory and voluntary sectors. The aim is for every child to have the support they need to:

- Be healthy
- Stay safe
- Enjoy and achieve
- Make a positive contribution
- Achieve economic well-being.

Some aspects of the programme are of particular relevance for bereaved children and families and the services supporting them: these include early intervention and prevention; support at times of transition, and support for parents. Children's Trust arrangements bring local authorities together with health, police, the voluntary sector, and other agencies to work in partnership to achieve children's outcomes. This gives greater opportunities for community based childhood bereavement services to be involved in local planning and service delivery. As the impact of bereavement cuts across all aspects of children's lives, it has been easy for agencies to see it as someone else's job: working together means that it should be seen as everyone's responsibility.

Beyond children's policy, the End of Life Care strategy makes provision for bereavement care and support which is 'particularly important for children facing and then coping with the death of someone important in their lives' (Department of Health 2008 p112).

The development of services in the UK

Current policy informs a compelling justification for childhood bereavement services. However, other stimulating factors have played an important part in encouraging service development in the UK over the last 15 to 20 years. In response to professional experience (Willis 2005) and to changing ideas about childhood and bereavement (Rolls 2007a), the hospice movement's expertise in supporting the dying and their families has been extended to children and young people. Other stimuli include an increase in knowledge about children and their parents' experiences of bereavement, the establishment of services such as Winston's Wish in Gloucestershire in 1992, which became a model for many other area based childhood bereavement services, and an increasing demand from families themselves for services (Willis 2005).

The present situation

Given the range of factors inspiring the development of services, it is not surprising to see just how diverse the sector is, revealed by a study of 108 services carried out by Rolls and Payne (2003 2004). Specialist services have emerged from various sectors: while 14% of the services in their study were solely dedicated to working with bereaved children, the vast majority were offered as part of the wider work of a host organization. Almost half of these were hospices: others included adult bereavement services and generic counselling services. This diversity is also reflected in the staffing make-up of services, 73% of which were using a mixture of paid staff and volunteers, who came from a wide range of professional backgrounds including counselling, nursing, social work, medicine, psychology, and play and art therapy.

Services typically offer a range of interventions, many of which are described in this volume. Direct support may be focused on the child or work with the whole family, and may be offered to individual children or families or in a group setting (Rolls and Payne 2004). Looking at eight case studies, Rolls and Payne (2004) identified eight main objectives underpinning the interventions. These were to:

- provide a secure place for exploration
- access unspoken and unconscious feelings
- help make sense of what had happened and how the users felt
- help users manage those feelings
- improve communication between family members
- create memory and story
- reduce feelings of isolation
- hold the possibility of hope for the future.

(Rolls and Payne 2004, p. 317)

Additional services are often offered to local professionals, including training, supervision, and signposting.

Restricted and open access services

A key distinction is often made between 'restricted' and 'open access' services (e.g. Willis, 2005). Restricted access services are usually offered to a particular group of children, often those bereaved through a particular cause, such as life-limiting illness. Twenty-nine percent – mostly hospice bereavement services– of the services in Rolls and Payne's study worked specifically with children related to a former user of the service who had now died. Restrictions can also be placed on how children and young people access help: almost three quarters of the services took referrals from either families or professionals, with 3% taking them from professionals only, 15% only accepting existing service users, and 10% taking referrals from families themselves only (Rolls and Payne 2003). We know little about how young people access services directly for themselves (Ribbens McCarthy with Jessop 2005).

By contrast, open access services (71% of Rolls and Payne's sample) generally offer a range of support services to children and young people whatever the type and circumstances of the death, the only restrictions on their services being the age of the child or young person, and the geographical area. The Childhood Bereavement Network in the UK maintains an online directory which currently holds details of 72 such services. It estimates that around 45% of local authority areas in England are only partly covered by an open access service, or not covered at all.

In areas without an open access service, there is often a difference in the support available to children and families bereaved through an anticipated death (e.g. cancer) and those that are unexpected (e.g. heart attack, road traffic accident). When a death is expected, information, guidance, and support before and afterwards is often available from an adult or children's hospice or palliative care team, although there are inequalities in access to specialist palliative care (National Audit Office 2008). Children and families bereaved through sudden death may find it much harder to access support both in the short and longer term. In the immediate aftermath, various professionals may complement support offered by family and friends: e.g. a faith leader, funeral director, hospital staff, or school staff. If the death was traumatic or violent such as through murder, suicide or road traffic accident, additional support may be offered by the police, hospital, Victim Support, social work teams, critical incident teams or a self-help group. If children later shows difficulties, they might be offered help from a school counsellor, educational psychologist, or in more severe cases, a referral to Child and Adolescent Mental Health services although waiting lists are often long and referral thresholds high (Willis 2005). Support may also be available from telephone helplines and email (see Stubbs 2009 this volume).

In essence, the provision of organised support is patchy. There is no one system for ensuring that bereaved families are provided with the information and guidance they might need to support their children. Even where services are available, funding is unreliable and services often face financial difficulties, despite diverse income sources (Rolls and Payne 2003). Jane Ribbens McCarthy's literature review suggests that young people who are already disadvantaged are both more likely to experience bereavement and multiple loss, and less likely to have organized support available to them (2005).

Co-ordinating the field

Many of these services developed independently and initially there was 'minimal national debate and no agreed standards or guidelines' (Stokes et al. 1999). Some coordination was needed and in 1998 the National Association of Bereavement Services launched a multi-agency collaborative project 'to improve the quality and range of bereavement support for children, young people and their families in the UK'. Collaboration with Marie Curie Cancer Care, a series of consultation events and funding from the Diana, Princess of Wales Memorial Fund resulted in the launch of the Childhood Bereavement Network in 2001, linking services and establishing a framework of standards for good practice in working with bereaved children and young people (www.childhoodbereavementnetwork.org.uk).

Now hosted by the National Children's Bureau, the Childhood Bereavement Network (CBN) continues to grow as a membership organization. Currently, over 300 organizations and individuals subscribe to CBN, endorsing the Belief Statement and Guidelines for Good Practice as a criterion of their membership.

Subscribers to CBN share a vision in which:

> all children and young people in the UK, together with their families and other caregivers, can easily access a choice of high-quality local and national information, guidance and support to enable them to manage the impact of death on their lives.

All subscribers to CBN have a role to play in realising this vision. CBN's own aims are to

- raise awareness of the needs of bereaved children, and the services available to them
- support our network of subscribers in their development and delivery of a range of high quality, accessible childhood bereavement services
- influence national, regional and local policy in the interests of bereaved children, young people, their families and other caregivers
- extend the capacity of the children's workforce to respond to the needs of bereaved children.

CBN produces a range of information for those setting up new childhood bereavement services or reviewing existing provision, distilling the expertise of subscribers in developing practice that is safe, fair, reflective, and sustainable (Penny 2005). Factsheets also provide suggestions on establishing the need for a service, raising funds, involving users in service development, and developing specific pieces of work with parents and carers.

An important aspect of CBN's activity is to synthesize and disseminate examples of good practice in working in particular fields or with particular groups of children and young people. The Diana, Princess of Wales Memorial Fund has recently funded such activity to develop approaches to working in schools, working with bereaved children and young people who are looked after by the local authority, and those who are living in secure settings. The Fund has also supported CBN as the national voice for the sector, adding value to the work of subscribers. The recent Grief Matters for Children campaign has called for appropriate support for all bereaved children and their families, wherever they live and however they have been bereaved, and sought to promote this through policy work and parliamentary lobbying.

Future challenges

Two key priorities for the UK childhood bereavement field over the next five years are to ensure that a range of services are available wherever bereaved children live, and however they have been bereaved, and that these services are robustly evaluated. Practitioners have long recognised the challenges of measuring childhood bereavement services' impact (e.g. Stokes et al. 1999) and a recent mapping of evaluations revealed 'an overwhelming, if cautious, consensus' among services for working together to develop a common set of evaluation tools including a national outcomes measure (Rolls 2007b p58). Incorporating the views of bereaved children, young people and their families, as well as developments in research and practice, this will strengthen the confidence in – and sustainability of – childhood bereavement services across the UK, helping to improve the quality of bereaved children and young people's lives.

References

Axford, N. (2008) *Exploring Concepts of Child Well-Being*. Bristol: The Policy Press.

Childhood Bereavement Network (2001) *Mission, Aims, Belief Statement and Guidelines for Good Practice*. London: National Children's Bureau.

Childhood Bereavement Network (2002) *A Death in the Lives of ...* London: National Children's Bureau.

Childhood Bereavement Network (2003) *You'll Always Remember Them, Even When you're Old*. London: National Children's Bureau.

Childhood Bereavement Network (2004) *It Will be Ok.* London: National Children's Bureau.

Childhood Bereavement Network (2007) *Grief Matters for Children: Campaign Briefing* London: National Children's Bureau.

Christ, G. (2000) *Healing Children's Grief: Surviving a Parent's Death from Cancer.* Oxford: Oxford University Press.

Currier, J.M., Holland, J.M., Neimeyer, R.A. (2007) The effectiveness of bereavement interventions with children: a meta-analytic review of controlled outcome research. *Journal of Clinical Child and Adolescent Psychology,* (**3**)2: 253–259.

Department for Children, Schools and Families *Every Child Matters Outcomes Framework* Available from http://publications.everychildmatters.gov.uk/default.aspx?PageFunction= productdetails&PageMode=publications&ProductId=DCSF-00331-2008 (accessed 26 January 2009).

Department of Health (2008) End of Life Care Strategy. London: The Stationery Office.

Dyregrov, A. (2008) *Grief in Children.* London: Jessica Kingsley Publishers.

Fauth, B., Thompson, M., Penny, A. (forthcoming) *Associations Between Childhood Bereavement and Children's Background, Experiences and Outcomes : Secondary Analysis of the Mental Health of Children and Young People in Great Britain 2004 data.* London. NCB

Harrington, R. and Harrison, L. (1999) Unproven assumptions about the impact of bereavement on children. *Journal of the Royal Society of Medicine,* **92**: 230–233.

HM Treasury (2003) *Every Child Matters* London: The Stationery Office.

National Audit Office (2008) *End of Life Care: A Report by the Comptroller and Auditor General.* London: The Stationery Office.

Penny, A. (2006) *A Guide to Developing Good Practice in Childhood Bereavement Services.* London: National Children's Bureau.

Prout, A. and James, A. (1997) A New Paradigm for the Sociology of Childhood? Provenance, Promise and Problems. In James, A. and Prout, A. (eds) *Constructing and Reconstructing Childhood.* 2nd edition. Abingdon, RoutledgeFarmer.

Ribbens McCarthy, J. (2006) *Young People's Experiences of Loss and Bereavement: Towards an Interdisciplinary Approach.* Berkshire: Open University Press.

Ribbens McCarthy, J. with Jessop, J. (2005) *Young people, bereavement and loss: disruptive transitions?* London: National Children's Bureau.

Rolls, E. (2007a) Containing Grief: *Ambiguities and Dilemmas in the Emotional Work of UK Childhood Bereavement Services.* Unpublished doctoral thesis, Department of Natural Sciences, University of Gloucester.

Rolls, L. (2007b) *Mapping Evaluations of UK Childhood Bereavement Services.* Cheltenham: University of Gloucestershire.

Rolls, L. and Payne, S. (2003) Childhood bereavement services: a study of UK provision. *Palliative Medicine,* **17**: 423–432.

Rolls, L. and Payne, S. (2004) Childhood bereavement services: issues in UK provision. *Mortality,* **9**(4): 300–328.

Rolls, L., and Payne, S. (2007) Children and young people's experiences of UK childhood bereavement services. *Mortality,* **12**(3): 281–303.

Sandler, I., Wolchik, S., Ayers, T., Tein, J-Y., Coxe, S., and Chow, W. (2008) Linking theory and intervention to promote resilience in parentally bereaved children. In Stroebe, M., Hansson, R., Schut, H., Stroebe, W. (eds) *Handbook of Bereavement Research and Practice*. Washington DC: American Psychological Association.

Stainton Rogers, W., (2004) Promoting better childhood: constructions of child concern. In Kehily, M.J. (ed) *An Introduction to Childhood Studies*. Maidenhead: Open University Press.

Stokes, J. (2004) *Then, Now and Always: Supporting Children as They Journey Through Grief: A Guide for Practitioners*. Cheltenham: Winston's Wish.

Stokes, J. (2007) Resilience and bereaved children: helping a child to develop a resilient mindset following the death of a parent. In Monroe, B. and Oliviere, D. (eds) *Resilience in Palliative Care: Achievement in Adversity*. Oxford: OUP.

Stokes, J., Pennington, J., Monroe, B., Papadatou, D., and Relf, M. (1999) Developing services for bereaved children: a discussion of the theoretical and practical issues involved. *Mortality*, 4(3): 291–307.

United Nations (1989) *Convention on the Rights of the Child*. New York: UN.

Willis, S. (2005) Work with bereaved children. In Monroe, B., and Kraus, F. (eds) *Brief Interventions with Bereaved Children*. Oxford: Oxford University Press.

Woodhead, M. (1997) Psychology and the Cultural Construction of Children's Needs. In James, A. and Prout, A. (eds) *Constructing and Reconstructing Childhood*. Abingdon: RoutledgeFarmer.

Worden, J.W. (1996) *Children and Grief: When a Parent Dies*. New York: Guilford Press.

Chapter 2

Theoretical perspectives: linking research and practice

Liz Rolls

Introduction

The word 'theory' 'sometimes seems to scare people, and not without good reason' (Craib 1992 p3) – a comforting thought as we embark on a chapter concerned with theoretical perspectives. There is an uneasy relationship between researchers and practitioners, and difficulty in linking research and practice that continues to be hard to reconcile. Nevertheless, as the chapters in this volume emphasize, working with bereaved children is a reflective and responsive activity that draws on different areas of knowledge, and involves an attuned receptivity to the complex psychological and social needs of individual children located in diverse contexts of loss. Furthermore, the increasing emphasis on evidence-based practice requires practitioners to justify their service provision and prove the efficacy of their actions. In this chapter, I consider theoretical perspectives in the context of childhood bereavement and services designed to support them, and explore the challenging and dynamic relationship between theoretical perspectives, research, and practice.

The nature of theory and theoretical perspectives

We all have theories and, on the basis of these, develop a broader hypothesis about life that frames our world view. Here, however, we are talking about theory in a way 'that is different from the everyday perception' (Alasuutari 1998 p164), enabling us to make sense of the problems of everyday life (Craib 1992) and stretching our understanding beyond the boundaries of the familiar world (Alasuutari 1998). Theories are generated through an individual's contemplation (for example, Karl Marx), but are also the goal of research, influencing how a phenomena is studied and underpinning its conduct. In the hypothetico-deductive mode of quantitative research, prior theory directs the processes of data collection, analysis, and interpretation. In the naturalistic paradigm of qualitative research, the move is from data towards new theory (Henwood and Pidgeon 1993).

Disciplinary knowledge

Theories are also informed by the discipline within which they are located, and many disciplinary perspectives inform the work of childhood bereavement practitioners, including:

- ◆ Anthropology: to understand cross-cultural variations in childhood bereavement and broader funerary practices;
- ◆ History: to understand bereavement practices over time in a particular social context, and how bereavement has been understood and researched over time;
- ◆ Psychology: to understand the impact of development and personality on childhood bereavement experience, and the effect of bereavement during childhood;
- ◆ Psychoanalysis: to understand the impact of unconscious processes and 'object relations' on the experience of childhood bereavement, and the place of childhood bereavement in unconscious adult life; and
- ◆ Sociology: to understand the socio-cultural aspects of grief and childhood bereavement, and the socio-linguistic aspects of how death and grief are spoken about.

In this chapter, I focus on the latter three perspectives.

Theoretical perspectives and world-views

During the 20th century, there has been a shift away from grand theory (such as those of Marx) towards a postmodern interest in the subjective experience of individuals (Denzin and Lincoln 1998). These differences manifest themselves in the different approaches of research as either:

- ◆ 'discovering/testing' a set of defined and pre-existing facts or laws about an objective world that is dispassionately uncovered in the research;
- ◆ 'generating' theory based on a view of the social world as contingent and fluid, which a researcher tries to understand; or
- ◆ evoking and embodying participation with, rather than abstract theorizing about, the stories of participants (Smith and Sparkes 2008).

This fluidity allows discourses to emerge (Henwood and Pidgeon 1993 p19), but also generates tensions and 'border skirmishes' that impact on the links between research and practice, and the 'use' practitioners can make of any given theory.

Theoretical perspectives: linking research and practice of working with bereaved children

Using a case study of a family bereavement, I now consider how different theoretical perspectives can provide insight and direction for practice.

The Case study

◆ *The death*

Susan (41) and Bill (44) were involved in a car accident. Bill, who was driving, was unhurt, but Susan was killed instantly.

◆ *Family life and history*

Bill and Susan lived in Essex with their three children: John (11) who recently moved to Senior School, Sally (8), and Jenny (5) who had just started school. Susan, an only child, grew up locally, but when she was 11 her mother died from breast cancer. Her father re-married and she has two half-brothers. She had a poor relationship with her step-mother and hardly knew her step-brothers who were still young when she left home. She has been at home with her children since their birth. Bill grew up in Wales where his parents, and his two brothers and their young families, still live. He runs his own business employing three members of staff.

◆ *Since Susan's death*

The three children attended the funeral, against the advice of Bill's parents, and returned to school shortly afterwards; each school was informed of their bereavement. Bill's parents stayed for four weeks, but returned home to take care of their other grandchildren. Seven months after Susan's death, the family are struggling – Bill is tired and lonely, and his relationships are suffering; John used to be outgoing but is now truculent; Sally tries to help as much as she can; and Jenny keeps asking when Mummy is coming back. Bill realizes they need help, and contacts a local childhood bereavement service.

Psychological theories and perspectives

From amongst a considerable number of psychological theories, two are relevant here.

Cognitive development

Each child is at a different developmental stage, which has an impact on their capacity to mourn. Christ (2000) identified developmental differences in children that were related to their eventual acceptance of the finality of death. This links with the view that the capacity to understand the concept of death as permanent, irreversible, inevitable, and universal comes with the children's cognitive maturation (Dyregrov 2008), and other factors, including differences in life circumstances (Wass 1991), their experience of death, religious beliefs, and what they are told (Stambrook and Parker 1987; Anthony and Bhana 1988-9).

These research findings alert practitioners to a number of features that it would be useful to explore. How is death spoken about in this family? What are their beliefs about life after death? What other experiences of death have the children had prior to their mother's? They also provide practitioners with useful information to discuss with Peter to enable him to understand that the 'fact' of their mother's death and its implications will need to be revisited over time, as the children reach more sophisticated levels of maturity.

Resilience: a theory of stress and coping

Resilience relies on a triad of factors: genetic and constitutional, including personal attributes such as positive self-concepts; a supportive family milieu, with close bonds to at least one family member; and the availability to parents and children of external support systems (Garmezy 1985; Werner 1995). Sandler et al. (2003) developed a bereavement-related stressors measure that included four categories: environmental changes; expectations of the child's behaviour; parental distress; and death reminders; the latter two, including parental demoralisation, having unique relations with children's mental health problems.

This perspective draws practitioners' attention to the value of understanding whether the parents were able to generate feelings of resilience in their children prior to the death of their mother, and it highlights some aspects of family history that it would be useful to explore. Each child may be 'resiliently' dissimilar as a result of their different personalities, ages and life experience. What kind of family environment had been fostered before Susan's death? What expectations were there on the children's behaviour, and how had each child been enabled to develop? To what extent had they been able to communicate their feelings to at least one parent or significant person, and what might be the implications if this is the parent who has died? Here, it is the mother who has died which correlates unfavourably with a greater risk of depression, especially for girls (Silverman and Worden 1993), and fathers are less likely to be able to use conversation in the wake of emotionally upsetting events (Dyregrov 2008). Both parents were isolated from their extended family, placing greater emphasis on the role of the nuclear family and the local community in fostering resilience. To what extent were the family embedded in this? Two of the three children have entered new communities just before their mother's death. Do their schools actively play a significant part in ameliorating their isolation (Rowling 2009 in this volume)? Moreover, Peter may be a demoralized parental figure struggling with feelings of remorse and the difficulties of managing his radically altered life.

Nevertheless, the Harvard Bereavement Study (Worden 1996) appears to indicate that most children are resilient to this stressful event, and some argue that there is no evidence of long-term effects of childhood bereavement (Ribbens McCarthy with Jessop 2005). However, there are debates about the links between adult psychopathology and childhood bereavement, and for more insight on this question, we need to turn to another theoretical perspective, that of psychoanalysis.

Psychoanalytic theories and perspectives

From amongst a considerable number of psychoanalytic theories, one is of particular relevance to this family.

Attachment theory

Attachment theory is a psychoanalytic object relations theory, developed by Bowlby (1980/1998), to account for the formation of close human relationships, and for what happens when separation occurs. He argued that an infant's survival depends on attachment to a close 'object', and that in instances of permanent loss such as bereavement, the feelings associated with separation – intense distress and behavioural responses – are triggered. He formulated a series of overlapping stages of grief involving: shock, yearning and protest, despair, and recovery. Building on this, Parkes' (1996) proposed that people progress through a number of phases before resolving their bereavement, and this has had a major influence on the work of adult bereavement services.

There are important insights to be gained from this theory that has implications for practice. Firstly, Susan's death constitutes an irrevocable separation invoking strong feelings of anxiety and distress in each of her children, associated with their own attachment style. Furthermore, Peter's demoralization may create further anxiety, provoking increased attachment-related behaviours. Practitioners can observe the children and wider family relationships, use these theories to understand each child's responses, and promote positive attachments to Peter and other adults – including themselves – as a secure, responsive figure. Secondly, whilst attachment and resilience theories have developed as two separate bodies of knowledge, attachment theory provides insight into the mechanisms underlying resilience (Atwool 2006), and more than 25 years of study have demonstrated the relation between secure attachment and the capacity to cope successfully with adversity, suggesting a link between attachment and subsequent ego resilience (Travis and Combs-Orme 2007). Interventions that support secure attachments will, therefore, contribute to increasing each child's resilience.

Sociological theories and perspective

Sociological theories locate grief and childhood bereavement within a socio-cultural, rather than an individual, context. However, rather than consider the implications for practice of the impact of the socio-cultural context as 'determinants' (Worden 1996) or 'moderators' (Neimeyer and Currier 2008) of an individual child's experience of bereavement, I discuss Mellor's (1993) theory of the 'sequestration of death' to show how broader cultural theories can contextualize childhood bereavement and the role of services.

The sequestration of death

Finding ways of coping with the intense threat posed by death has been an essential part of human society (Seale 1998). However, this threat has been exacerbated in the developed world by the loss of religious belief and collective rituals, resulting in the potential to 'open up the individual…to the dread of personal meaninglessness' (Mellor and Shilling 1993 p421). One solution to this threat is to suppress knowledge of this reality through the avoidance or denial of the experience and the organization of death (Mellor 1993; Mellor and Shilling 1993), into privatized cultural practices and organizations such as hospices, funeral services, and bereavement services. Children's experience of bereavement is not, therefore, solely mediated by their own disposition and the social relations and context that surround the immediate individual and their family, but is set within a culture that has increasingly devised social defences against the insecurity and chaos of death. However, the hiddeness of death from everyday life, and the loss of mourning practices and rituals has made the position of children increasingly precarious (Rolls 2008).

This theory links to practice in two ways. Firstly, it situates the bereavement of this family in a wider cultural context, and raises questions to explore about their own beliefs, practices and rituals: how meaningful are they to them? How are they shared inter-generationally, and what conflicts might arise if they are not? Until recently, the women or children in some communities have not attended funerals, and this may have been the case in Peter's parents' family tradition. It also provides an account for the difficulties people have in responding to the bereaved and, in the case here, raises questions about how relatives, friends, and other important social groups are able to respond to the children. How comfortable are they at 'naming' the reality of death, and facing the painful recognition of these children's fractured storylines (Brown and Addington-Hall 2008)?

Secondly, it provides a cultural, as opposed to a psychological, account for the rise and increasing place of childhood bereavement services in the landscape of UK services. Cultural anxiety about children's bereavement has been sequestered into a 'specialist' domain of 'experts', whilst at the same time, these services are a response to the vacuum created by the loss of ritual, the deep social anxiety about childhood bereavement, and cultural attempts to hide the reality of death from children (Rolls 2007a). Nwoye (2005) argues that bereaved people in Africa are never left in the dark about what is expected of them or what to expect from the culture (Rolls 2008). In listening to children's stories and attempting to meet the needs of bereaved children, services are filling this cultural vacuum, creating a symbolic community into which bereaved children are able to situate themselves, and through which to create a more resilient narrative of their experience (Rolls 2008).

In providing an alternative socio-cultural rationale for their existence, this account brings two benefits. Firstly, it enables services to situate their struggles for recognition and funding and the increasing demands being placed on them for evidence of their worth, within this wider cultural context. Secondly, it argues that services are not just passive *reproducers* of culture. Through their contribution to transforming cultural beliefs and attitudes towards bereaved children, services are becoming *producers* of culture (Rolls 2007a). Their increasing cultural importance – as an ecological niche in which children are enabled to face the reality of death and develop a narrative of their bereavement experience – provides a useful counterpoint to the focus on 'outcomes' of children's bereavement as a static concept, rather than as a dynamic experience within the context of their social relations, themselves set within a wider cultural context.

Issues in linking research and practice

This chapter has shown how theoretical perspectives can be linked to, and enhance, practice, and it has raised three key issues that I will discuss further.

The applicability of particular theory/research

A number of theories have been developed for adults and, over time, there has been a shift in emphasis to more psycho-social models such as Stroebe and Schut's (1995) 'dual process' model and Klass et al's (1996) theory of 'continuing bonds'. However, whilst there are theories upon which services draw that try to understand the nature and impact of childhood bereavement in the short- and long-term (Worden 1996; Christ 2000; Dyregrov 2008), there has been little theorizing of childhood bereavement in a way that is similar for adults, nor is there an understanding of children's grief from their perspective. As a result, in many service settings, adult-based theories are adapted for work with children (Rolls and Payne 2004, 2007), raising questions about their applicability.

In addition, there are issues concerning the quality of any study/meta-analysis and the underlying assumptions that are important to consider; as Fonagy (2008) asks: do researchers study care with care? For example, in relation to outcome research, there are often unasked questions about whose outcome it is and for whom it is positive – the child, parents, clinician or service purchaser (Fonagy et al. 2002), whilst to date in the UK, there are no agreed outcomes for child-hood bereavement to which services can make a contribution (Rolls 2007b). Fonagy (2004) argues that, with the greater appreciation that psychiatric disorders of adulthood are rooted in abnormalities already observable in childhood or adolescence, child and adolescent psychotherapy research of the future will have to be more firmly rooted in developmental psychopathology. In more recent years, the idea of enhancing resilience has influenced service practice and provided a level of justification for it. This attention – in the absence of clear outcomes and longitudinal studies – to the preventative strategy of enhancing individual resilience, and strengthening the social systems surrounding a bereaved child, may well be the most appropriate.

Nevertheless, theories and research provide practitioners with a basis for decision making, and a number of questions can help assess the applicability of any theory/research to practice, including:

◆ How applicable is the theory/research to this child/family/situation, and how 'valid' is it?

◆ Do I know enough about the theory/research AND the child/family/situation to use it in making decisions about interventions?

◆ What would it help the child/family to know about this theory/research? Is it appropriate for me to share this and, if so, with whom?

◆ In what ways does this theory/research NOT apply?

The changing and contestable nature of theory

As well as the applicability of theory to practice, there are also issues concerning the fluid nature of theory itself. As a system of ideas, there are no 'true' theories that fully account for the experience of loss, and the emotions, experiences, and cultural practices that characterize grief and mourning (Payne et al. 1999); rather, theories grow and develop over time [see Small (2001)]. Furthermore, theories arise and are elaborated within disciplinary perspectives, even if these may come to be challenged [for example, Seale (2003) and Craib (2003)].

Theories may also be misunderstood or misinterpreted. Fraley and Shaver (2008) argue that Klass et al's (1996) thesis of continuing bonds 'involves a caricature of Bowlby's views' (2008 p748), and Small (2008 p153) argues that 'simply to talk about letting go and moving on ... is the way critics of Freud précis his position ... [which] ... does not do justice to the idea of resolution presented by Freud ...' There are many reasons for this including academic rivalry, but two reasons are of interest. Firstly, there are cultural differences between disciplines whose underlying assumptions and world views mean it can be hard to understand the perspective within which the theory was created. Secondly, there are cultural differences between countries and the social policy contexts in which bereavement, children, interventions, and research are situated. Much of the research that influences understanding of childhood bereavement and the work of UK services comes from the US where, as well as differences in cultural attitudes and social norms with respect to both children and bereavement, there are significant differences in the funding of health and welfare services, and in cultural narratives. This raises questions about its transferability and about how childhood bereavement is conceptualized; is it a discrete medical problem, or a life event occurring in the dynamic context of a particular history to which meaning is attributed (Ribbens McCarthy 2006)?

Linked to this, is the question of how the outcome of bereavement is conceptualized. Frank (1995) identified a typology of illness narratives – *restitution*, *chaos*, and *quest* – and these have been used to consider the narratives of people with a range of conditions. Myers (2002) argues that the *restitution* narrative, the dominant illness narrative in the US, is problematic; the reluctance to give up hope for a cure, implicit in this narrative, may result in a lack of information or misinformation about end-of-life care, and compromises crucial end-of-life tasks and the possibility of transforming hope for a cure to a hope for quality of life until death. For this, the *quest* narrative, with its model of journey, would be a more fitting one to adopt, but there is a cultural resistance to adopting alternative narratives because to do so calls into question the positive and optimistic North American assumptive world (Myers 2002). In relation to childhood bereavement, is there an underlying assumption in the US of the 'restitution' of children to their pre-bereaved 'state' (Christ 2000), that contrasts with the quest metaphor exemplified in UK service names [*Jeremiah's Journey*], professional literature [*Then, now and always* (Stokes 2004)], and evaluation studies (McIntyre et al. 2007)? Is the *quest* narrative more in harmony with the objectives, common to UK childhood bereavement services to: help children make sense of what had happened, create memory and story (a narrative), and hold the possibility of hope for the future (Rolls and Payne 2004)? And if so, how can the applicability of research generated in an alternative social policy and narrative culture be considered?

Challenges in introducing and using theory and research in practice

Despite these reservations, the use of theory/research is crucial in informing practice; indeed, practitioners are already doing so (Rolls and Payne 2004).

However, introducing theory/research into practice is a challenging enterprise for three reasons. Firstly, working with bereaved children means that practitioners draw on a considerable number of theories from a range of disciplines, each of which are characterized by a burgeoning volume of literature. How can practitioners access, read, and evaluate theory and research which, although a vital task, is time-consuming? Secondly, if a theory or research finding does not appear relevant, it will not be incorporated into practice. Researchers and practitioners can judge the value of theory/research using the following questions:

- Does it provide an account to which service users and practitioners can relate? Does it 'speak' to their experience?
- Is it helping practitioners address the complex issues they face?
- Is it asking the right questions from their point of view, or from the view they have come to learn that children and families hold?
- In the case of outcome research, is it using the services' own criteria by which to judge them? Are these active and dynamic – concerned with learning, adaptation, and meaning – rather than passive and static?
- Does it capture the productive process in which the sorrow of life is faced? Is it in the service of children in their fight for resources?

Thirdly, there may be a lack of shared values, or a privileging of some theories over others. Individual practitioners are located in, and draw upon, a disciplinary base that frames their world view and informs the practices through which they provide support, but there are a variety of disciplinary perspectives amongst practitioners working within, and across, services, as well as across other services with whom they work. Introducing theory and research into practice is partially the responsibility of a reflective practitioner, but it also involves organizationally supportive strategies that might not be forthcoming, and may generate 'clashes of discourse'; a problem also arising between researchers/methodologies and practitioners.

Lastly, there is the issue of 'clinical lore' (Walter 1999). Reflective practice relies on a contemplative consideration of the practitioner's work, actions, motives, and thoughts in relation to others, and in relationship to literature (Johns 2004). However, it is not only other academics who misinterpret theory. In the process of 'clinical lore', practitioners transmute and solidify theories in a move from theory as 'insight' to theory as 'prescription', for which the misinterpretation of Freud's meaning of 'letting go', and the intensification of Parkes' (1996) phases of bereavement into a fixed sequence, are examples.

Concluding remarks

This chapter has explored the challenging and dynamic relationship between theoretical perspectives, research and practice. What can be concluded is that each of these make different assumptions about, and focus on different aspects of, bereavement, children, and society. As a result, there are different consequences that result from using any theory or research finding, and each will address the diverse dimensions of the bereavement experience of children. In the UK, membership organisations such as the Bereavement Research Forum (www.brforum.org.uk) provide opportunities for researchers and practitioners to discuss these theory-research-practice issues. With limits to research- and service-funding, what remains a challenge is the generation of theories and research that have relevance for UK-based practice.

References

Alasuutari, A. (1998) *An Invitation to Social Research*. London: Sage.

Anthony, Z. and Bhana, K. (1988-9) An exploratory study of Muslim girls' understanding of death. *Omega*, **19**: 215–227.

Atwool, N. (2006) Attachment and resilience: Implications for children in care. *Child Care in Practice*, **12**(4): 315–30.

Bowlby, J. (1980/1998) *Attachment and Loss, Vol. 3: Loss, sadness and Depression*. London: Pimlico. First published in 1980 by London: Hogarth Press.

Brown, J. and Addington-Hall, J. (2008) How people with motor neurone disease talk about living with their illness: A narrative study. *Journal of Advanced Nursing*, **62**(2): 200–208.

Christ, G.H. (2000) *Healing Children's Grief: Surviving a Parent's Death from Cancer*. Oxford: Oxford University Press.

Craib, I. (1992) *Modern Social Theory: From Parsons to Habermas*, 2nd Edition. Hemel Hempstead: Harvester Wheatsheaf.

Craib, I. (2003) Fear, death and sociology. *Mortality*, **8**(3): 285–295.

Denzin, N.K. and Lincoln, Y.S. (1998) Introduction: Entering the field of qualitative research. In Denzin, N.K. and Lincoln, Y.S. (eds) *The Landscape of Qualitative Research: Theories and Issues*, pp.1–34. Thousand Oaks: CA: Sage.

Dyregrov, A. (2008) *Grief in Children: A Handbook for Adults*, 2nd Edition. London: Jessica Kingsley.

Fonagy, P. (2004) Psychotherapy meets neuroscience: A more focused future for psychotherapy research. *Psychiatric Bulletin*, **28**: 357–359.

Fonagy, P. (2008) *Studying Usual Care with Care: The Example of MBT*. Keynote address at the UK Council for Psychotherapy conference From research-based practice to practice-based research. February, King's College, London.

Fonagy, P., Target, M., Cottrell, D., Phillips, J. and Kurtz, Z. (2002) *What Works for Whom? A Critical Review of Treatments for Children and Adolescents*. New York: Guilford Press.

Frank, A. (1995) *The Wounded Story-teller: Body, Illness and Ethics*. Chicago: University of Chicago Press.

Fraley, R.C. and Shaver, P.R. (2008) Loss and bereavement: Attachment theory and recent controversies concerning "grief work" and the nature of detachment. In Cassidy, J. and Shaver, P.R. (eds) *Handbook of Attachment: Theory, Research and Clinical Applications,* pp. 735–759. New York: Guilford Press.

Freud, S. (1917) *Mourning and Melancholia.* London: Hogarth Press.

Garmezy, N. (1985) Stress-resistant children: The search for protective factors. In Stevenson, J.E. (ed) *Recent Research in Psychopathology,* pp. 96–117. Oxford: Pergamon Press.

Henwood, K. and Pidgeon, N. (1993) Qualitative research and psychology. In Hammersley, M (ed) *Social research: Philosophy, Politics and Practice,* pp. 14–32. London: Sage.

Johns, C. (2004) *Being Mindful, Easing Suffering: Reflections on Palliative Xare.* London: Jessica Kingsley.

Klass, D., Silverman, P.R. and Nickman, R.B. (1996) *Continuing Bonds, New Understandings of Grief.* Washington, DC: Taylor and Francis.

McIntyre, R., Kennedy, C. Worth, A. and Hogg, R. (2007) *Evaluation of a Support Service for Children and Families Facing the Loss of a Parent From Cancer.* Final Report to Macmillan Cancer Support. Edinburgh: Napier University.

Mellor, P.A. (1993) Death in high modernity: The contemporary presence and absence of death. In Clark, D. (ed) *The Sociology of Death,* pp.11–30. Oxford: Blackwell.

Mellor, P.A. and Shilling, C. (1993) *Modernity, Self-identity and the Sequestration of Death.* Sociology, 7(3): 411–431.

Myers, G.E. (2002) Can illness narratives contribute to the delay of hospice admission? *American Journal of Hospice and Palliative Care,* 19(5): 325–330.

Neimeyer, R. and Currier, J.M. (2008) Bereavement interventions: Present state and future horizons. *Grief Matters,* Autumn, 18–22.

Nwoye, A. (2005) Memory healing processes and community Intervention in grief work in Africa. *Australian and New Zealand Journal of Family Therapy,* 26(3): 147–154.

Parkes, C.M. (1996) *Bereavement: Studies of Grief in Adult Life,* 3rd Edition. London: Routledge.

Payne S., Horn, S. and Relf, M. (1999) *Loss and bereavement.* Open University Press: Buckingham.

Ribbens McCarthy, J. with Jessop, J. (2005) *Young People, Bereavement and Loss: Disruptive transitions?* London: National Children's Bureau for the Joseph Rowntree Foundation.

Ribbens McCarthy, J. (2006) *Young People's Experiences of Loss and Bereavement: Towards an Interdisciplinary Approach.* Maidenhead: Open University Press.

Rolls, E.M. (2007a) *Containing Grief: Ambiguities and Dilemmas in the Emotional Work of UK Childhood Bereavement Services.* Unpublished PhD thesis, University of Gloucestershire, UK.

Rolls, L. (2007b) *Clara Burgess Charity Project 'Mapping Evaluations of UK Childhood Bereavement Services: Final Report,* University of Gloucestershire, UK.

Rolls, L. (2008) The ritual work of UK childhood bereavement services. In Earle, S. Komaromy, C., and Bartholomew, C. (eds) *Death and Dying: A Reader,* pp. 175–183. Sage/Open University: London/Milton Keynes.

Rolls, L. and Payne, S. (2004) Childhood bereavement services: Issues in UK provision. *Mortality,* 9(4): 300–328.

Rolls, L. and Payne, S. (2007) Children and young people's experience of UK childhood bereavement services. *Mortality,* **12**(3): 281–303.

Rowling, L. (2009) Loss and grief in school communities. In Monroe, B. and Kraus, F. (eds) *Brief Interventions with Bereaved Children,* 2nd Edition, pp. 147–160. Oxford: Oxford University Press.

Sandler, I.N., Wolchik, S.A., Davis, C., Haine, R.A. and Ayers, T.S. (2003) Correlational and experimental study of resilience for children of divorce and parentally bereaved children. In Luthar, S.S. (ed) *Resilience and Vulnerability: Adaptation in the Context of Childhood Adversities,* pp. 213–240. New York: Cambridge University Press.

Seale, C. (1998) *Constructing death: The Sociology of Dying and Bereavement.* Cambridge: Cambridge University Press.

Seale, C. (2003) Commentary: Fear, death and sociology: A response to Ian Craib. *Mortality,* **8**(4): 388–391.

Silverman, P.R. and Worden, J.W. (1993) Children's reactions to the death of a parent. In Stroebe, M., Stroebe, W., and Hansson, R. (eds) *Handbook of Bereavement: Theory, Research and Intervention,* pp. 300–306. Cambridge: Cambridge University Press.

Small, N. (2001) Theories of grief: A critical review. In Hockey, J., Katz, J., and. Small, N. (eds) *Grief, Mourning and Death Ritual,* pp.19–48. Buckingham: Open University Press.

Small, N. (2008) Theories of grief: A critical review. In Earle, S., Komaromy, C., and. Bartholomew, C. (eds) *Death and Dying: A Reader,* pp.153–158. Sage/Open University Press: London/Milton Keynes.

Smith, B. and Sparkes, A.C. (2008) Narrative and its potential contribution to disability studies. *Disability and Society,* **23**(1): 17–28.

Stambrook, M. and Parker, K.C.H. (1987) The development of the concept of death in childhood: A review of the literature. *Merrill Palmer Quarterly,* **33**: 133–157.

Stokes, J. (2004) *Then, Now and Always: Supporting Children as They Journey Through Grief: A Guide for Practitioners.* Cheltenham: Winston's Wish.

Stroebe, M. and Schut, H. (1995) *The Dual Process Model of Coping with Loss.* Paper presented at the meeting of the International Work Group on Death, Dying and Bereavement, Oxford, 29 June.

Travis, W.J. and Combs-Orme, T. (2007) Resilient parenting: overcoming poor parental bonding. *Social Work Research,* **31**(3): 135–149.

Walter, T. (1999) *On bereavement: The Culture of Grief.* Buckingham: Open University Press.

Wass, H. (1991) Helping children cope with death. In Papadatou, D. and Papadatou, C. (eds) *Children and Death,* pp. 11–32. New York: Hemisphere.

Werner, E. (1995) Resilience in development. *Current Directions in Psychological Science,* **4**: 81–85.

Worden, J. (1996) *Children and Grief: When a Parent Dies.* New York: Guilford Press.

Chapter 3

Bereavement, young people and social context

Jane Ribbens McCarthy

Introduction: meanings-in-contexts

The lives of young people are embedded in networks of relationships and social contexts and circumstances. It follows, therefore, that we cannot understand their bereavement experiences in the round without paying full attention to such social and cultural issues. And while the significance of such social contexts makes itself felt through the meanings that individuals, including children, give to their experiences, social contexts in turn help to shape meanings. Contexts are thus not 'external' to individuals, but are inextricably *interlinked* with meanings, and in this regard it can be useful to think about 'meanings-in-contexts' to indicate how deeply each is implicated in the other.

Decisions made by bereavement researchers and practitioners in themselves constitute part of the contexts shaping the meanings of 'childhood bereavement'. In this regard, the predominant focus on parental and sibling deaths renders some forms of bereavement much more visible than others. But this professional and research focus may only be partly justified by reference to evidence, since we know that deaths of close friends as well as parents and siblings can be important for mental health outcomes (Green 2005) and young people themselves may refer to a much wider range of relationships when asked about significant losses they have experienced (Harrison and Harrington 2001). Indeed, if we look beyond the contexts of minority western societies, the meanings of particular deaths in children's lives may be different again. Among young people living in the Central African Republic, for example, deaths of parents may not necessarily be included amongst those losses which individuals list as causing most grief (Hewlett 2005).

For the remainder of the chapter, however, I will focus on the research evidence we have available to us, rooted as it is in particular cultural understandings and empirical work based in European and New World societies.

Social issues in children's bereavement experiences

If we attend to young people themselves talking about their experiences of bereavement, social relationships emerge as key themes (Ribbens McCarthy 2006). The availability of social support may thus be a key factor to consider (Silverman and Worden 1992; Green et al. 2005). In terms of personal networks, including friends, peers, wider kin relations and other significant adults, it seems that such personal ties and contacts can significantly shape children's experiences of bereavement, but may work in quite opposing directions, for good or ill. The presence of close friends, for example, is the category of people most often mentioned by young people as being helpful (Gray 1989; Rask et al. 2002). In this regard, it is relevant to consider general research suggesting that close communications between parents and young people may often be experienced in quite complex and ambivalent ways (e.g. Gillies et al. 2001), while talking to friends may be experienced as more straightforward.

However, social contacts are not necessarily helpful in themselves, since peers may also be involved in name-calling, bullying etc. (Cross 2003; Worden 1996). Even where peers are not actively destructive, children and young people may find that their relationships suffer as their peers struggle to know how to react, with the potential for feelings of isolation developing among bereaved children (Murphy 1986; Worden 1996). Loneliness and a sense of difference may indeed persist into adulthood as a long-term implication of childhood bereavement (Holland 2001; Servaty and Hayslip 2001), constituting a potentially important long term consequence of experiences of death in the early years. This perhaps emphasizes the potential importance of peer group support, whether informally or more formally facilitated, in schools or elsewhere.

Beyond personal support, social contexts also crucially provide young people with clues about how to understand and manage life events. The social contexts important here include immediate personal networks, but also extend to broad political circumstances, as in the case of children bereaved through the Troubles in Northern Ireland (McNally 2005). The ways in which such broad cultural-societal-political contexts impinge on children's bereavement experiences, framing their meanings in particular ways, and perhaps linking to wider community and personal traumas, has received little research attention. However, the broader literature on childhood trauma draws our attention to the ways in which minority western cultural assumptions underpin research on children's resilience in different contexts (Ungar 2008), and may also unhelpfully frame interventions with children experiencing traumatic events in situations of political conflict (Boyden 2003).

The significance of contexts in outcomes over time

Within the broad quantitative research evidence concerned with childhood 'risk', some studies consider whether the death of a parent during childhood is statistically associated with an increased probability of a variety of unwelcome outcomes. The evidence of such a direct link is complex and contradictory (reviewed in Ribbens McCarthy 2006), but there are a number of potential ways to understand this complexity, including: the possibility that different individuals react in opposite directions in ways that cannot be picked up in large scale data sets; the importance of understanding childhood bereavement not just as a single event but alongside other difficult life experiences; and the possibilities afforded by more sophisticated multivariate analyses to consider parental death alongside a variety of other aspects of children's lives. Multivariate analyses have rarely been undertaken concerning the outcomes of parental death during childhood, but such analyses of the impact of parental divorce/separation may provide useful food for thought about childhood bereavement. Such studies point to the importance of individual differences, but also to broader issues of social and material contexts.

Various aspects of family relationships have thus been identified as a key consideration for the outcomes of both divorce/separation (see, for example, Hetherington 2003; Dunn 2008) and parental death (Worden 1996). Firstly, it may be important to take account of processes over time, in terms of family relationships (particularly parental conflict, and level of ambivalence) prior to the divorce/separation or death as such. Secondly, the quality of the relationship with the remaining parent has been shown to be crucial for children's well-being after divorce/separation (Hetherington 2003; Dunn 2008) and after parental death (Gersten et al. 1991; Haine et al. 2006). Furthermore, there may be quite opposite effects going on (Sutcliffe et al. 1998), with some parentally bereaved children becoming closer to their surviving parent and others becoming hostile (Worden 1996). Thirdly, family dynamics and relationships may also be important to consider more broadly, with the bereaved young person exercising their own agency and input into these processes (Demi and Gilbert 1987). Here, too, there may be opposite tendencies occurring in different families, with siblings sometimes found to be particularly helpful *or* unhelpful after parental or sibling deaths (Worden 1996), while the well-being and 'competence' of other surviving family members may be important for support *or* its absence (Gersten et al. 1991). Some family relationships may deteriorate to 'extreme alienation' (Gray 1989) or outright abuse (Cross 2003) after parental bereavement.

Throughout all these processes, the gender of the child and the gender of other survivors may interact in complex ways (Ribbens McCarthy 2006).

Death of a mother, for example, may be more disruptive of everyday life, while death of a father may have greater significance for household income and resources (which in itself may vary by social class) (Corden et al. 2008). Finally, in terms of other social relationships with adults beyond the immediate household, we know little about the importance of grandparents after a parental death, but the presence of a close relationship with a grandparent or another adult has been found to mediate the impact of divorce/separation (Hetherington 2003).

It will be apparent from this brief overview, that family relationships, particularly in terms of the well-being of the surviving parent, have received some useful research attention in the literature on childhood bereavement. However, what is generally overlooked is the ways in which such family processes may be *inter-linked* over time with other features of social and material context more widely. Worden (1996), for example, found that a 'passive coping style' exhibited by the surviving parent was important for parentally bereaved children's emotional and behavioural difficulties. He also discusses how parental coping style relates to other stresses, such as financial worries, health problems, larger family size, younger age of surviving parent. Nevertheless, he does not discuss potential links between such stressors, parental coping style and the consequences for children. In other words, perhaps some parents develop a passive coping style as a result of feeling overwhelmed by lack of resources and a history of difficult events. Similarly, Worden points to the significance of affluence for reducing the likelihood of bereaved children being 'at risk', and he also presents evidence of the importance of the number of changes in daily life over time (such as moving house, changing school) for the quality of family relationships and for parental depression. However, he does not discuss whether more affluent households are better placed to avoid too many such changes in daily life.

The presence or absence of such resources – in terms of material circumstances and social contexts – may be understood to reflect the broad patterns of inequalities and class in society, constituting features of social structure. Indeed, the likelihood of experiencing the death of a parent or sibling may itself be related to social class, since we know that social class, patterned by geography and locality, is still a major factor in mortality rates (Mitchell et al. 2000). Bereavement patterns may also be different among refugee children. Furthermore, as raised above, affluence may work as a protective factor in many interconnected ways, and it is important to note the finding of Sandler et al. (1997) that relatively minor additional stressful events may affect children's adjustment to a single major negative life event like parental death.

Overall, then, broad structural issues such as social class, gender and race, have implications for both individual and family experiences of childhood bereavement. As Marris observes, 'Inequalities of power affect both vulnerability to bereavement and the ability to recover from it' (1996 p118). An important aspect of this may be the ways in which childhood adversities may be clustered within particular families. Experience of such multiple difficulties (including multiple bereavements) has been shown to be more important than the experience of a single problematic life event (such as parental death) in putting children at risk of serious negative consequences (e.g. Green et al. 2005). In turn, such clustering of adverse experiences is likely to be related to structural disadvantages e.g. in terms of social class or race (Newman 2002).

Conclusion

While such quantitative research analyzes regular patterns in children's lives, it is necessary to remember that individual lived experiences are messy and complex, and survey findings cannot be directly applied to individual children. Such methodologies may usefully identify broad trends, about which groups of individuals might most need help and intervention, but they may struggle to capture the ways in which children make sense of, and give meaning to, their lives and experiences. In this regard, it is also important to research individual life course histories to see how individual and social processes occur interactively over time. In this chapter, I have sought to delineate some of the ways in which social contexts of a variety of types are a crucial part of this complexity, but I have also argued that we need to understand how far social context and child are not separate features but are integrally bound up together. This applies not only to the more immediate social contexts of family, personal networks and locality, but also to those broad features of social context – such as social class, gender and race – that we might refer to as social structure. These are all features of social lives that refer to patterns and systematic processes that occur across a range of individual experiences. But these are not just features of an 'external' social reality, they also enter in the consciousness of individuals. In the present discussion, they might impinge, for example, on the extent to which an individual child repeatedly experiences the world as unsafe and unpredictable, such that a significant bereavement is taken as one more, perhaps crucial, indication that life is not to be trusted.

The evidence presented here points to the central importance of acknowledging these connections between personal, interpersonal, localized, societal, cultural and political issues if we are to understand the responses of individual children to the death of someone significant to them. While academics and researchers may endeavour to find ways of encompassing this complexity, professionals and practitioners working with individual children may struggle with the 'broader' social issues that may seem outside the scope of their interventions. But while it may thus be frustrating and even painful to consider how far interventions with individual children and families may be limited in their scope in the face of broader structural issues such as multiple disadvantage and material inequalities, I believe it is nevertheless vital for social contexts, in all their manifestations, to be included in the picture. While it is crucial to attend to the meanings by which individual children actively seek to make sense of their life experiences, wider social, cultural and political contexts are also reflected in individual consciousness itself.

References

Boyden, J. (2003) Children under fire: challenging assumptions about children's resilience. *Children, Youth and Environments*, **13**(1). http://www.colorado.edu/journals/cye/13_1/Vol13_Articles/CYE_CurrentIssue_Article_ChildrenU. Accessed on 24 March 2009.

Corden, A., Hirst, M., and Nice, K. (2008) *Financial Implications of Death of a Partner* (Working Paper No. ESRC 2288). York: University of York.

Cross, S. (2002) *'I Can't Stop Feeling Sad': Calls to Childline about Bereavement*. London: Childline.

Demi, A.S., and Gilbert, C.M. (1987) Relationship of Parental Grief to Sibling Grief. *Archives of Psychiatric Nursing*, **1**(6): 385–391.

Dunn, J. (2008) *Family Relationships: Children's Perspectives*. London: One Plus One.

Gersten, J.C., Beals, J., and Kallgren, C.A. (1991) Epidemiology and preventive interventions: parental death in childhood as an example. *American Journal of Community Psychiatry*, **19**: 481–498.

Gillies, V., Ribbens McCarthy, J., and Holland, J. (2001) *'Pulling Together: Pulling Apart': The Family Lives of Young People Aged 16–18*. London: Joseph Rowntree Foundation/Family Policy Studies Centre.

Gray, R.E. (1989) Adolescents' perceptions of social support after the death of a parent. *Journal of Psychosocial Oncology*, **7**: 127–144.

Green, H., McGinnity, A., Meltzer, H., Ford, T., and Goodman, R. (2005) *Mental Health of Children and Adolescents in Great Britain*. Basingstoke Hants: Palgrave Macmillan.

Haine, R.A., Wolchick, S.A., Sandler, I.N., Millsap, R.E., and Ayers, T.S. (2006) Positive parenting as a protective resource for parentally bereaved children. *Death Studies*, **30**: 1–28.

Harrison, L., and Harrington, R. (2001) Adolescents' bereavement experiences. Prevalence, association with depressive symptoms, and use of services. *Journal of Adolescence*, **24**(2): 159–169.

Hetherington, E.M. (2003) Social support and the adjustment of children in divorced and remarried families. *Childhood: A Global Journal of Child Research*, **10**(2): 217–253.

Hewlett, B.L. (2005) Vulnerable lives: the experiences of death and loss among Aka and Nganda adolescents of the Central African Republic. In Hewellet, B.L. and Lamb, M.E. (eds) *Hunter-Gatherer Childhoods: Evolutionary, Developmental and Cultural Perspectives*. (pp. 322–342). New Brunswick, New Jersey: Transaction Publishers.

Holland, J. (2001) *Understanding Children's Experiences of Parental Bereavement*. London: Jessica Kingsley.

Marris, P. (1996) *The Politics of Uncertainty: Attachment in Private and Public Life*. London: Routledge.

McNally, D. (2005) *The Influence of Social Contexts on Bereavement: A Qualitative Study of Adults Bereaved During Childhood and Adolescence Due to the Northern Ireland Troubles*. Unpublished Masters dissertation in Social Research Methods, Open University, Milton Keynes.

Mitchell, R., Dorling, D., and Shaw, M. (2000) *Inequalities in Life and Death: What if Britain were More Equal?* Bristol: Policy Press/Joseph Rowntree Foundation.

Murphy, P.A. (1986) Parental death in childhood and loneliness in young adults. *Omega-Journal of Death and Dying,* **17**(3): 219–228.

Newman, T. (2002) *Promoting Resilience: A Review of Effective Strategies for Child Care Services*. Exeter: University of Exeter.

Rask, K., Kaunonen, M., and Paunonen-Ilmonen, M. (2002) Adolescent coping with grief after the death of a loved one. *International Journal of Nursing Practice*, **8**: 137–142.

Ribbens McCarthy, J. (2006) *Young People's Experiences of Loss and Bereavement: Towards an Inter-disciplinary Approach*. Buckingham: Open University Press.

Sandler, I.N., Wolchik, S.A., MacKinnon, D., Ayers, T.S., and Roosa, M.W. (1997) Developing linkages between theory and intervention in stress and coping processes. In Wolchik, S.A. and Sandler, I.N. (eds) *Handbook of Children's Coping: Linking Theory and Intervention* (pp. 3–40). New York: Plenum Press.

Servaty, H.L., and Hayslip, B. (2001) Adjustment to loss among adolescents. *Omega-Journal of Death and Dying*, **43**(4): 311–330.

Silverman, P.R., and Worden, J.W. (1992) Children's reactions in the early months after the death of a parent. *American Journal of Orthopsychiatry*, **62**: 93–503.

Sutcliffe, P., and Tufnell, G. (1998) The relevance of tears: reconstructing the mourning process from the systemic perspective. In Sutcliffe, P. Tufnell, G. and Cornish, U. (eds) *Working with the Dying and Bereaved*. Basingstoke Hants: Macmillan.

Ungar, M. (2006) Resilience across cultures. *British Journal of Social Work*.

Worden, J.W. (1996) *Children and Grief: When a Parent Dies*. New York: The Guilford Press.

Chapter 4

Swampy ground: brief interventions with families before bereavement

Gillian Chowns

In a book about children's bereavement this chapter is different because its focus is on working with children *before* a death. It will draw on findings from recent research conducted by both child and adult co-researchers and will use a number of case examples to illustrate the key principles – many of which will no doubt be familiar to readers.

The context

Pre-bereavement work has to contend with one major and unique issue – uncertainty. However distressed the bereaved child is, she is dealing with certainty; something important has happened. This also applies to the worker. But supporting children in a family where a parent or grandparent is seriously ill is like wading through a swamp that has been sown with land-mines. There is precious little solid ground. What there is may be likely to blow up in our face. We cannot always be certain of the outcome – whether this father will survive, or how long we may have to work with the child, so judging how we should pace our work is difficult. We may have just a few days, or perhaps several months; our first visit may also be the last or we may see child, parent or both half a dozen times. Nevertheless, as the following case-studies demonstrate, effective intervention does not necessarily require long-term therapeutic work. While our work usually reflects the experience of the sick person – that there is never enough time – it also reflects another truth of palliative care: that it is perfectly possible to make a difference even when time is limited, and often precisely *because* time is limited, as the following situation demonstrates.

First meetings – the Broad family

Mother was already seriously ill when I first met her and her husband. It seemed likely that there might be a month or so to work with their two daughters, aged eight and ten, and I planned the first session accordingly, aiming to establish some rapport and trust, to explain who I was and how I might help, and to offer them some choice about whether and how we might work together. I also hoped to clarify both what they *knew* and *felt* about their mother's illness. The visit went well and I felt I had achieved most of the objectives. I then formulated a clear plan for the next visit. But it was postponed because the mother was admitted to the local hospice that day. She died a week later and my plan was obsolete. (That is not to say that plans are not useful, just that we must always be willing to amend or abandon them in the light of the situation that presents itself rather than the one that we have anticipated.) Nevertheless, the foundation stones of the work were in place, even though the focus had shifted from supporting the children through their mother's illness to offering bereavement support. The girls – and their father – knew that help was available, that they could choose when and how to access it, and that the meaning that their loss had for them would be recognized and respected. Thus, although the referral had left us very little time to work together, it had still been possible to establish the core conditions of trust, respect and choice for an effective intervention.

- Establish trust
- Check understanding as well as knowledge
- Offer options and agree a possible way forward

Listening – the Taylor family

Roy and David Taylor were teenage brothers whose mother was terminally ill. Teenagers are generally recognised to be hard to engage, and boys more difficult than girls. So the combination of gender and age was not encouraging. In addition, it was their father who instigated the referral. However, after the initial meeting, the boys agreed to a second visit. Offered the choice of being seen individually (my own private preference) or together, they chose the latter, and I had two sessions with them before their mother died. I began by suggesting that, although I knew the main facts from their father, they might like to tell me the story in their own words. And that's what they did. What *I* did, almost exclusively, was to listen. The value of this simple 'narrative' approach was threefold. First, it enabled them, perhaps as never before, to put the pieces together, to establish a chronology, and to make some limited sense of events. Secondly, it enabled them to articulate some of their beliefs and meanings about the experience. Thirdly, they were able to explore, challenge, and build on each other's differing memories, perceptions and concerns. Contrary to all the family's expectations, 14-year-old David was almost as vocal as the more confident Roy. Both boys admitted to being surprised about this, while I wondered to myself whether David would have said anything at all if I had followed my own instincts and seen him separately.

In this situation the ability to listen, to offer some prompts (sparingly), to take the boys seriously, and to acknowledge in the beginning that they had some choices about how they used the help that they had not asked for, was sufficient. More than a year later, in response to a researcher's interview, one said, 'It was good doing it before [Mum died] rather than after ...... it was in a big part of our brain, it was on our minds all the time. ...... I wasn't as upset when she actually died as I thought I would be because I had come to terms with it then, and if I had the counselling after ... I might have been more upset'. So gender and age are important – but they are not insuperable.

- Listening to the story is often the most important thing we do
- Acknowledge that everyone will experience the story differently – there is no one truth.

Differentiation – the Howarth family: pace, level, and age

Alison Howarth, whose story highlights the positive and negative outcomes of outliving her prognosis by many months, had two children. Stuart, aged 14, had behavioural difficulties and was a weekly boarder at a Special School, while his sister Emma, bright and articulate, was 11. They were each struggling with the roller-coaster of mother's illness. The nature of my work with Emma was different from that with Stuart. Emma needed information about the disease, its consequences and outcomes, but she also needed the opportunity to debate its implications for her – coming up to puberty, self-conscious about her developing breasts and only too well aware of her mother's mastectomy. A number of our conversations were essentially debates about body image, although we did not use that language. Work with Stuart was much more task-oriented, concrete, and present rather than future-focused. Nevertheless, Stuart had a more realistic understanding of the situation than either parent realised, as shown after an explosive family row, when Dad lost control and shouted, 'Don't you know she's going to die?' Stuart was able to give a good account of what that meant. 'I know she's ill and she won't get better and she'll go on getting iller, but it isn't like she's going to die tomorrow or next week, it could be a month or more'. His basic understanding was good, his emotions and behaviour much less mature. On the four or five occasions I met with him, either at home or school, I con- sciously tried to pitch my approach largely – though not exclusively – at his emotional age. Often angry at life, he frequently complained that 'it's not fair', and I was able to use this as a *motif* for our work. Although the concept of fair- ness was an abstract, we could work together on what was fair to expect from each family member. Used to a system of rewards and punishments, Stuart was comfortable in negotiating a 'fair' contract with his family about how much he helped around the house, how much special time he got with his mother and how frequently he could ring to check on things at home during his weekly absence. A week was a long time in his life and I needed to adjust my approach accordingly. With Emma, I could work more swiftly and reflectively, recognizing that she was much older than eleven most of the time, but that occasionally she needed to be more like a seven year old. Thus the pace of the work took into account the children's (multiple) ages. But it also needed to take into account the likely dying trajectory (Mansell Pattison 1997) of their mother, levels of awareness (Glaser and Strauss 1965) and anticipatory grief (Lindemann 1944). These concepts are familiar to professionals and may enable us to face the uncertainty that both the family and we experience. But the reality for Stuart and Emma was that they went to school each day not knowing whether their mother would still be at home in the afternoon, or whether she would have had another fall and another hospital admission. They knew their mother would die soon, but after every crisis she was still there. It became hard for them to live in this limbo. For them, those last few months were an eternity. They did not know what 'anticipatory grief' meant, but they knew it was harder to be close to Alison. For that chronologically brief but emotionally extended period, it was important that the worker did not model that detachment and distance but demonstrated a willingness to stay with them in their pain, listen to their anger and acknowledge their weariness and fear. When uncertainty and exhaustion combine, the reliable presence of someone genuine, warm, and empathic (Egan 1990) can be a useful, short-term, counterbalance.

- ◆ Emotional maturity may be more important than chronological age
- ◆ Identify and work with the child's concerns, at the child's intellectual level
- ◆ Being (there) may be as important as doing

Ethical issues

Short-term interventions are liable to criticism from those who argue that effective intervention requires sustained, long-term, intensive work. Others criticize the grief and counselling 'industries', with Walter (1994) having characterized its proponents as 'grief police', peddling a one-size-fits-all approach, inappropriate for a post-modern society, and Harrington and Harrison (1999) suggesting that interventions may do more harm than good. Yet there is increasing evidence that skilled short-term work before a death can be beneficial for both child and family. Writers such as Jewett (1994) and Christ (2000) offer a sound theoretical base for practice, while recent research, discussed below, involving child service-users has highlighted the key issues that they themselves identify (Chowns 2009).

Children's rights

In the UN Convention on the Rights of the Child (1989), articles 12 and 13 clearly set out the right of a child to be informed, consulted and involved in any 'matters which affect their well-being'. For the first time, and applicable to all cultures, there is a public, global acknowledgement that children should not only be seen but also be heard – that they are capable of forming their own views and that those views must be considered carefully. However, in Western society, there is a deep ambivalence about children. We have extended the period of childhood, in terms of education and economic dependence, into the late teens; yet we have also shortened it drastically, as we turn childhood into a consumer experience and target children as mini-adults, selling them life-style and success through the latest 'must-have' trainers, clothes or computer games. We are both pro- and anti-children in almost equal measure. On the one hand, we see them as innocent, vulnerable and in need of protection and, on the other hand, we see them as dangerous – hanging round on street corners, out of control, and in need of discipline and containment (Beresford 2002).

Our own participative inquiry, in which a group of nine children met together to research their own experience of living with seriously ill parents and to produce a film on the subject, was predicated on Articles 12 and 13. The children (Jack and Becky, Rachael, Laura and Megan D, Laura C, twins Gemma and Natalie, and Ellis) identified the themes to be researched, conducted interviews with each other and exercised editorial control over what went into the film they were making; the process showed that the children were potentially competent to decide what was right for them, capable of identifying what types of support they needed and entitled to have their views heard and respected. This led to a revisioning of the models of childhood currently seen in the UK and the formulation of a new, more respectful model, that of the Able Child-Citizen (Chowns 2006) (see Fig. 4.1).

Key findings

It was clear from this research that children unequivocally prefer to be informed and involved. They wish to be told the truth as fully and as soon as possible. Delay and deception, for whatever motives, are experienced as destructive of trust. Children seek support and understanding rather than protection and prevarication. Nevertheless, the research also demonstrated clearly that children are capable, competent individuals who are active, reciprocal family

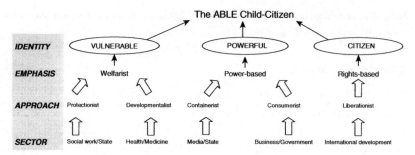

Fig. 4.1 The ABLE Child-Citizen.

members, not only carefully selecting coping strategies, but also endeavouring to support and understand their parents.

I now consider a number of the key findings.

Impact of cancer

Facing the life-threatening illness of a parent brings a sense of isolation and the uncertainty about their parent's and their own future is all-pervasive.

It became obvious that creating and maintaining the self in relation to cancer was an ongoing challenge for the children. A basic, powerful and unresolved conflict was located in the tension between their own perception and presentation of themselves as competent, able individuals and the more traditional emphasis on the vulnerability of children in society generally. They wanted their abilities and expertise to be recognized, and were frustrated when that recognition was lacking.

Nevertheless, this sense of self, and confidence in self, was seriously threatened by the advent of their parent's illness. The children characterized it as turning their world upside down, undermining both their abilities and their relationships. They found it harder to maintain their normal selves, and its disabling effects on their parent was mirrored in their own experience:-

'Cancer takes your real life away … takes your confidence away'

Rachael

It was experienced as affecting their functioning on all levels, including the intellectual, because it was all-pervasive and inescapable, cluttering up the very pores of existence:

'When cancer clogs your life … your brain capacity gets clogged with pollution'

Laura C

Not knowing whether or when the cancer would return increased this sense of helplessness, and several of the children spoke of their frustration and fear in living with this uncertainty; cancer, even when treated, was characterized as a ghost that continued to haunt their waking moments. On the other hand, although cancer was beyond their control, being made more helpless by the well-meaning actions of adults was taken very personally. Both Laura and Ellis experienced their parents' decision to delay telling them of the diagnosis as unhelpful, marginalizing them in the family and undermining their perceptions of themselves as competent and significant.

Agency and empowerment

Children will consciously adopt specific strategies in order to gain some control over the family situation.

In the journey to empowerment, Warren (1997) supports Rapoport's analysis (1970), which emphasizes the importance of a strengths-based philosophy, ascribing difficulties less to the incompetence of the individual (child) and more to the institutional and societal structures which prevent the display or acquisition of competence and power. Our group's experience reflected this dilemma and revealed a number of strategies for managing this tension.

Once they knew about the diagnosis, the children demonstrated considerable agency in their choice of what they shared, with whom they shared, and when they shared both information and feelings. They adopted conscious strategies for managing their situation, preserving their sense of self and maintaining a sense of normality in the face of a disease that was often out of control, and a family life that had become chaotic, unpredictable, and unsafe. The choice of whom to tell was based primarily on trust and intimacy, with most of the youngsters telling only their closest friends:

'I can talk about it to one person I can trust – Rachael'.

Becky

These selected friends could be trusted to handle the information sensitively and with respect, whereas others, though they might not laugh about it, might take it less seriously and, equally worryingly, spread it around the school. Clearly, it was important to the children to be able to retain some sort of control over the information, even though they knew they could not exercise control over the cancer itself.

Knowing what it was not safe to say led to other strategies for staying in control. For example, many of the children either did not trust well-meaning enquirers or did not trust themselves to stay in control of their feelings, and dealt with this by a strategy of dissembling:

'To get them off your back, say that she's fine'.

Rachael

Truth-telling

Children prefer truth to prevarication

Every member of the group wanted not only to be told the truth but to be told the whole truth:

> 'Tell us the truth, tell us everything. Don't hide it, it makes it worse, freaks you up. Tell us exactly what's going on'.

Twins

Knowing the truth was not easy but was clearly preferable to being kept in the dark; Megan's advice to parents was

> 'Tell your kids everything that's going on or they'll not know nothing. Supposing you go into hospital – then they'll not know nothing'.

Ellis summed up much of this discussion succinctly:

> 'Children should be told what they want to know. They should be told the truth and nothing but the truth'.

There was a general consensus about the timeliness of telling. Everyone wanted to be told immediately, and cordially disliked delay and secrecy.

> 'If you're told late, you just feel you've done something wrong..'

Rachael

> "Mum was diagnosed on my birthday – she didn't tell me till the Saturday'.

Laura C

> 'Tell us straightaway, or we're more upset'.

Rachael

Foretelling

Mixed views on talking about the future

Telling, in the sense of talking out loud about whether someone might die, was acknowledged as risky by some of the group, because it might become foretelling – 'it might make it happen'. However, others, including Ellis, aged 15, disagreed with the premise entirely, and felt that talking about the possibility made it easier to accept.

Not talking and telling

Communication is complex and multi-layered

A significant coping strategy for some of the research group was 'not-talking'. Putting on a smile, being non-committal, and avoiding the subject of their sick parent were ways of 'not-talking' and allowed them to remain in control of both the conversation's content and their own emotions. Laura D, the middle of the three D siblings, also made a useful distinction between talking and telling, saying at one point that talking with friends was helpful because it did not involve talking about cancer, but later making it clear that there was just one person for whom she broke her rule about telling.

'I've only told one friend'

Laura D

Despite her reluctance to talk either on camera or off, Laura D challenged our assumed understandings of talking by her careful distinctions between 'talking to' (having friends), 'talking about' (discussing) and 'telling' (informing others about the illness).

Adult: 'Do you talk to friends when you're stressed?'
Laura: 'Not really'
Adult: 'Is it easier to avoid (the subject)?'
Laura nods.
Even the act of speaking the word 'Yes' is best avoided; she resorts to body language only, explaining much later that '*I don't like drawing attention to myself*', a sentiment shared in part by Becky who also admitted that she didn't like talking '*in front of other people*'. For them, it was not necessarily that cancer was difficult to talk about, but that it was difficult to talk in the public arena.

Megan also did not find it easy, but was able to talk more readily about not finding it easy to talk! Furthermore, she could acknowledge the value of talking to others undergoing the same experience:

'This project's very good ... we're making new friends, talking to people going through the same situation ... brilliant ... having someone to talk to'.

Ellis, the oldest of the co-researchers, tended to be economical with his words, but he made them count:

'I bottle everything up inside, then a couple of times a year it just overflows' (sweeping gesture with his arms).

Both the palliative care and counselling literature have tended to assume that those who talk readily find it relatively easy, but this is not necessarily a safe assumption. Laura C commented in one of the later sessions that she preferred not to talk about someone dying because she feared it becoming a reality. To the challenge by an adult that she was often the first person to raise an issue, she explained:

'It's easy to talk about it here, 'cos we're all going through round about the same thing but talking to the actual person who is ill, that's hard'.

So, not talking might have several explanations – embarrassment, shy personality, magical thinking, or it might be dependent on which person it was to whom one was *not- talking*. It was usually a deliberate, considered decision.

Unfortunately, many adults, including professionals, tend to assume that if children do not talk they do not care or are not worried. However, this was emphatically not the case for our co-researchers:

> Laura C: [You can't ask your parent] 'Are you going to die, when are you going to die, how is it going to happen, will I be there?'
> Adult: 'But these are things you'd quite like to talk about?'
> Laura C: 'Well in a way, in a way, not'
> Adult: 'But they are things you are thinking about?'
> Laura C: 'Yes!'

Thinking, as opposed to talking, often reflected the ambivalence at which Laura hinted in the above exchange. Holding two opposing thoughts in juxtaposition was a coping strategy, and the children often demonstrated a mature awareness of multiple and inconsistent positions: Gemma commented that *I didn't exactly expect him to get better, but I hoped he would,* while Laura C explained, *You want to hide away, but you want someone to find you.*

Working with the messiness of practice

In the research setting, we worked, and acted, with the revised model – that of the Able child-citizen – as dominant, but in much of palliative care practice, the earlier models may well persist, and parental wishes and rights may conflict with those of the children.

Some parents will be reluctant to involve a palliative care social worker, even though teachers and health professionals may have well-founded concerns about the child's need for support. Other parents will assure a worker that their child is keen to be seen, but it quickly emerges on a first visit that he has little understanding of who that worker is or what they do, and has been given no choice in the matter of meeting them. The parent's *need* to help their child, however well-intentioned, has overridden the child's *right* not only to consent but to give an *informed* consent to the meeting. And even when all this has been negotiated satisfactorily, and the parents have initially demonstrated an openness and honesty, things may change as death approaches.

The following situation illustrates the parental struggle to maintain openness and to respect the capacity and competence of children – competence that was respected in our research project, but that, for very well-intentioned reasons, may not be forthcoming in the home setting. It also offers some pointers in helping the parent to reconsider their approach.

Helping parents to help their children

The Andrews family had been impressive in their willingness to face the likely loss of Martin, father of Jenny and Todd and husband to Elaine. Now that Martin was deteriorating noticeably, Elaine was, typically, anxious to think ahead to what would happen when he died. She wondered if she should send the children away to her own mother 'when it gets really close'.

She thought it might be sensible to get the children back into school as soon as possible after the death, as 'it would be better than hanging round the house'. She supposed that Jenny, aged seven, was too young to go to the funeral, but that Todd, at nine, was probably old enough. She was a little surprised by the question, 'What do Jenny and Todd think?' but it provoked a fruitful discussion, in which I highlighted the very sensitive way she had responded to their different needs and understandings so far, and how consistent she had been in checking out at each stage how much they understood, how much they wanted to know, and how involved they wanted to be in Martin's care. Her child-centred approach had worked well to date, so maybe there was no need to change it now. Elaine was able to admit, somewhat ruefully, that she had uncharacteristically not considered the children's wishes. Our discussion then moved on to ways of raising these issues with the children, but was interrupted by the arrival of Todd in the sitting room. In a three-way conversation between us, Todd revealed how he was worried about being teased at school because 'When Dad dies, they will call me a bastard, because I won't have a Dad any more'. Between us, Elaine and I were able to help Todd work out a plan. Todd thought he himself would want to tell his best friend when his Dad died, but that he would like his class teacher to tell the class – 'but when I'm not there'. A question about who he might want to talk to, if he got very upset, elicited the answer, 'Mrs Taylor', the class helper. Later, after I'd left, Elaine was able to have a similar conversation with Jenny, who was much less certain about what she wanted. The discussion with Todd, however, had enabled Elaine to suggest some options to Jenny, so that together they agreed an acceptable plan. On my next visit, Elaine was keen to tell me how supportive the school had been when she had contacted them. She was pleased and relieved to have a plan in place – but quickly acknowledged that the children might easily change their minds when it came to the actual event. She could apply the same caveat to the discussion she was planning to have with them about attending the funeral. She was no longer so focused on protecting them from what she had thought would be an unsuitable and distressing experience. She now wanted to support them, and was able to recognize their right to be involved, if that was their choice. Involvement, to her, had meant simply attending, but as she talked about what

Martin wanted (cremation) and the hymns he had chosen in advance, I was able to ask the same basic question again, 'What will Todd and Elaine want (to contribute)?' Although Elaine did not feel strong enough to talk in detail about the funeral with the children at this stage, the fact that we had been able to think through the issues meant that when Martin eventually died the children were involved and included as much as they wanted to be. Both of them chose to put a favourite item in the coffin; each had a suggestion for some music to be played during the ceremony, and a memory about their father that the minister could share with the congregation. Todd was clear that he not only wanted to go to the funeral but that he wanted to see his father's body at the undertaker's. Jenny was less sure; she said she would go with the others, but she wouldn't go in and see the body. Elaine said that was fine, and that her grandmother would wait with her outside the room. In the event, Jenny surprised them by electing to go in just as they were ready to leave. Elaine followed the same principle with the funeral, taking account of the children's wishes, but offering the option for them to change their minds right up until the service itself. This time, she had prepared a cousin of hers, well-known to the children, to go with them if either became so distressed that they didn't want to stay. The fact that (at some emotional cost to herself) she had taken them both to the crematorium a few days before the funeral and had painstakingly explained what happened in the service, including when the coffin would disappear behind the curtains, meant that both Todd and Jenny were better able to cope; they both stayed throughout the service. Elaine faced some criticism from some of her relatives but was sustained by Todd's comment, 'All those other people were there, but they weren't family like we are, I needed to be there for Dad'.

The importance of memories

In the weeks before Martin's death, the children and I had talked about some of the special memories they had of their father. Sometimes it was a family outing that they recalled, sometimes it was a mannerism of his, or a saying he was fond of. Some of these 'favourite things' were captured in the workbook that Jenny and I used, but Todd had not wanted to do one. Using his computer for the same end, however, worked very well. Todd liked lists, and was happy to compile a long list of all his father's favourite things – food, colours, TV programmes, etc. After Martin died, the workbook and the computer file served as prompts for Todd and Jenny, enabling them to hold on to precious memories. While some of the adults around them avoided Martin's name, as if he had never existed, the children had their own treasure store which they could 'activate' as and when they needed.

It is not only memories that need preserving; for children, as for adults, possessions may carry a significance way beyond their material value. Children may be hesitant about asking for something belonging to the dying parent, so it may be helpful for the worker to raise the issue. For some families, a memory box in which significant items are kept has pride of place; for Todd, wearing his father's watch was all that mattered. As he confided in me, 'It smells of him, and that makes me sad, and happy'.

- ◆ Facilitate parent-child communication
- ◆ Gently challenge untested assumptions
- ◆ Encourage families to involve children in funeral plans – and respect their choices
- ◆ Make it clear that it is OK to change your mind at any time
- ◆ Find ways of preserving memories of the dead parent.

Firm foundations

Both social work and health care ethics require us to consider not only how we approach our work but to be clear about the evidence which may or may not underpin what we do in the messy world of real practice.

The literature on childhood bereavement is, by definition, retrospective – even when the interviews focus on life before the parent died, the young person is recalling it as a past event with the benefit of hindsight, in full awareness that death was the outcome. It is likely that the previous dearth of pre-bereavement research mirrored the practice situation – that professionals found this area frightening. There may be three reasons for this. First, its very uncertainty – its 'swampy' nature – makes *us* uncertain of our abilities and skills. Secondly, the combination of children and death is both powerful and disabling. We instinctively reject it as not natural; it challenges our notions of fair play, and the innocence of childhood. Our instinct, like that of so many parents, is to protect the children – and possibly ourselves. We fear making things worse. Just as many parents from the best of motives avoid talking to their children about such painful issues, so many researchers may have avoided this area for the same reasons. Ethical concerns about intruding on grief, raising levels of anxiety, making children fear the worst may be understandable or even legitimate, but the consequence is that until recently they have been marginalized and disempowered; their voice is not heard. Thirdly, the area may just be too personally uncomfortable. Staying alongside the distress of children is difficult; it confronts us with both our own remembered childhood and also with our own mortality – another uncomfortable combination.

For these, and maybe other reasons, pre-bereavement groups such as my own team's 'Video Project' are much rarer than bereavement groups. Yet, as Christ acknowledges in her Foreword to this book's first edition, (pv) children 'experienced their highest levels of anxiety and depression *before* the parent's death' (my italics) and both her own large scale study, which researched families both pre- and post-death (Christ 2000) and the research discussed above, strongly indicate that preparatory work before the death, can be of immense value.

Palliative care in general has been vulnerable to the charge that there is no base for its effectiveness. Part of the problem, of course, is agreeing what constitutes an evidence-base. Whether it is either feasible or desirable to apply positivistic notions of measurement to the individual kaleidoscope of experiences, meanings and values that make up a child's journey through life is debatable. But the recent research projects highlighted above offer some useful models and theories that provide a solid foundation for our work. They may guide, though not prescribe, our interventions. And if we strive to be reflective practitioners, and remember to reflect both on, and in, action (Schon 1987) we will be open to recognising the strengths within children. As Alderson (1995) and Barnard (1999) have suggested, children are not simply passive recipients of skilled adult professional intervention, but are active participants in their own lives, marshalling their own peer-based support networks, seeking out and processing information, selecting strategies, and essentially exercising control. We therefore need to respect their competence even as we attempt to offer support; we are not the all-powerful deus ex machina working on the blank canvas of another human being, but are subject to social, political and cultural contexts and ultimately to the main actor, the child, who will herself judge whether she needs or wants to work with us.

Last words

Children whose parents are seriously ill present particular challenges. Their status in society is disputed; their competence and understanding undervalued. Their rights and needs are often in conflict with those of their parents. Their future is uncertain, for they do not know when they will join the ranks of the bereaved. Yet, effective work with these children rests on a few, well-known, simple precepts. Our role is not to become part of the problem by increasing their dependence on us, but rather genuinely to empower them to find their own way.

In the DVD made by our own young people's group (Chowns et al. 2007), there are two clear messages from all the children: the first is 'Tell us the truth' and the second is 'Don't tell us that you know how we feel – you don't. We're all different'. We need to respect those differences. If we are able to hold on to those guiding principles of honesty and respect, choice and control, while accepting difference we shall stand a good chance of negotiating both the minefields and the swamp.

References

Alderson, P. (1995) *Listening to children*. Barkingside: Barnados.

Barnard, P., Morland I., and Nagy J. (1999) *Children, Bereavement and trauma*. London: Jessica Kingsley.

Beresford, P. (2002) Maturity needed. *Community Care,* July 11, 2002.

Chowns, G. et al. (2007) *"No- You Don't Know How We Feel" (DVD)* gpatgc@aol.com

Chowns, G. (2006) *"No – You Don't Know How We Feel"; Researching the experience of Children Living with Life-Threatening Parental Illness, Through Collaborative Inquiry.* Unpublished PhD thesis. University of Southampton.

Chowns, G. (2009) End of life care discussions - but not in front of the children? *End of Life Care,* **3**(1): 42–47.

Christ, G. (2000) *Healing children's grief.* New York: Oxford University Press.

Egan, G. (1990) *The Skilled Helper.* California: Brooks Cole Publishing.

Glaser, B. and Strauss, A. (1965) *Awareness of Dying.* Chicago, IL: Aldine.

Harrington, R. and Harrison, L. (1999) Unproven assumptions about the impact of bereavement on children. *Journal of the Royal Society of Medicine,* **92**: 230–233.

Jewett, C. (1994) *Helping Children cope with Separation and Loss.* Boston: BT Batsford.

Kissane, D.W. and Bloch, S. (2002) *Family Focused Grief Therapy.* Buckingham: Open University Press.

Lindemann, S. (1994) Symptomatology and management of acute grief. *American Journal of Psychiatry,* **101**: 141–148.

Mansell Pattison E. (1997) *The Experience of Dying.* New Jersey: Prentice Hall.

Monroe, B. and Kraus, F. (2005) *Brief Intervention with Bereaved Children* (1st edition), Oxford: Oxford University Press.

Rapoport, R. (1970) Three dilemmas of action research. *Human Relations,* **23**: 499–513.

Schon, D. (1987) *The Reflective Practitioner.* San Francisco, CA: Jossey Bass.

United Nations (1989) *Convention on the Rights of the Child.* Geneva: United Nations.

Walter, T. (1994) *Revival of Death.* London: Routledge.

Warren, C. (1997) Family support and the journey to empowerment. In Cannan, C. and Warren, C. (eds) *Social Action with Children and Families.* London: Routledge.

Chapter 5

Family assessment[1]

Julie Stokes

How families experience bereavement

'The family' is often a key context for determining the development and well-being of children who grow up within a family. As such, the family is a crucial component of any assessment of a bereaved child or young person who may be in need of a bereavement service. The assessment also needs to extend to other key relationships and contexts, for example, school, peers, and so on. Each family is different. Everyone will experience their grief differently: this will be shaped by their individual, family, cultural, social, and religious beliefs and means that no two deaths are ever mourned in exactly the same way.

During the early weeks and months after a death, the family unit is inevitably fragile, vulnerable, and seemingly frozen in time. Shapiro (1994) describes grief as a crisis which becomes interwoven with family history, and has a dramatic effect on how the family develops as a new unit—'a family in developmental crisis'. Each family will struggle to stabilize after a death, and its first priority in managing the crisis is to work towards a stable equilibrium within which the family can try to move forward. 'With a developmental approach that considers the family as a unit of distinct yet inextricably interconnected members, we can help families survive and grow while bearing the burden of death and loss' (Shapiro 1994).

Assessing the family as a whole provides insight into the way a child is related to as part of a family group. This information is central to understanding the ways in which a family is able to safeguard and promote the well-being of the child, and whether there are aspects of family life and relationships which compromise its capacity to do so.

A family assessment provides a vehicle for observing and describing what the practitioner can learn from talking with families and from their

---

[1] Adapted from 'Preparing for the journey'. pp. 48–67 (Stokes, J.A. (2004).
In *Then, now and* always: *supporting children as they journey through grief – a guide for practitioners*. Cheltenham: Winston's Wish).

interaction together. The technique used can be a positive intervention in itself; promoting clarity and understanding of how individuals within a family are experiencing the bereavement. It is a way of learning about families in a detailed, relatively objective, evidence-based profile of family competence, considering family strengths alongside difficulties (Glaser et al. 1984). Although this chapter will focus on the process of conducting an assessment in the family home, the same principles apply for a telephone or an outpatient assessment.

Aims of the assessment

The assessment aims to establish:

+ the impact of this particular death
+ for this particular family
+ at this particular time
+ living in this particular community.

In making the assessment, the key determinants of grief identified by Parkes and Weiss (1983) need to be considered:

+ the nature of the attachment
+ mode of death
+ historical antecedents
+ personality variables
+ social variables
+ rituals
+ concurrent stressors

The purpose of the home assessment is to:

+ build trust so that the family feels 'safe' working with the organization/counsellor
+ give information about the possible interventions so that the family can make an informed decision about future involvement
+ collect information about the person who has died and attempt to understand how the death has affected the child(ren), other members of the family, and the wider community
+ find out about the child's knowledge and understanding of death
+ demonstrate how we can safely talk to children about death and grief
+ allow the family to talk about the death in as much detail as they want: this can be the first opportunity they have had to do this, and is often a therapeutic intervention for the family

- evaluate the degree of resilience/vulnerability observed in the family
- assess whether the services on offer could enhance resilience/reduce vulnerability
- assess whether referral onto another agency is also appropriate
- draw up an action plan: this may include some time to think and reflect before deciding to participate in the suggested intervention.

Who is involved in the assessment?

At Winston's Wish (a community child bereavement programme) it is our usual practice for two practitioners to make the initial visit; this helps to ensure that each family member has a chance to share their story individually. It also enables the practitioners to be confident that they themselves have reached a shared understanding of the key issues relevant for this particular family.

The following case study summarizes some key issues that emerged from a home assessment of an adolescent boy and his grandmother.

Case study: Ben (14)

A referral was received from Ben's head teacher. Ben has been having significant problems at school and was currently excluded following a mobile phone theft and abusive behaviour.

His mother died 3 years ago in a car accident and he now lives with his maternal grandmother.

A phone call to his grandmother (Anne) gathers additional information; Ben has a stepsister (Jemma) aged 8. Ben had lived with his mother and his stepfather until his mother's death. Since then Ben has experienced a difficult relationship with his stepfather who was driving the car at the time his mother died. Given the tense family dynamics, it is negotiated that the first assessment involves meeting with Ben and Anne at home with a view to making contact with Ben's step family (if appropriate) after that initial meeting.

A home assessment was arranged. Ben met with a practitioner on his own and his grandmother also had an opportunity to share her story with another practitioner. At the end everyone met up to discuss the best way forward. The assessment revealed that Ben harbours some strong feelings of regret and resentment over his mother's death. He explained that he had planned to join them on the car trip but refused to go shopping at the last minute and stayed with a neighbour playing computer games.

It transpires that Ben believes his stepfather was driving dangerously and that the accident would not have happened if he had been there. The accident happened at the beginning of the school holidays and it resulted in Ben moving out of his family home to live with Anne and a change to his planned secondary school move. He moved 10 miles away and lost regular contact with friends and his sister. He said his grandmother had threatened to put him in a home if his behaviour didn't improve. He admitted to stealing money to buy drugs to escape from it all.

The assessment identified a number of issues which would be addressed during a series of six individual sessions using a cognitive behavioural approach. The service also looked at facilitating links with his stepfather and sister with a view to enabling the family to attend a residential weekend group intervention. Ben also gave his permission for the assessment report to be sent to his year tutor, so the school had a clearer understanding of the issues he was facing following his mother's death.

Skills needed by practitioners

The ability to understand the influence of a variety of interconnecting factors is an essential skill in carrying out a systemic assessment. Grief is a deeply shared family developmental transition, involving a crisis of attachment and a crisis of identity for family members, both of which have to be incorporated into the on-going flow of family development. The assessment process needs to take stock of all facets of the family system both before and after the development has been interrupted by death and grief. A structured assessment pack is used to ensure a systemic framework is adopted for all assessments. (Stubbs et al. 2006). However, experienced practitioners will inevitably use their 'clinical intuition' (Greenhalgh 2002) to decide the order of questions rather than rigidly following the order of questions in the pack. Such clinical intuition makes sure they engage with family members and allows individuals to work in their own time and to their own priorities. Although confidence will come from having listened to the experiences of many bereaved families, practitioners will need to develop a set of skills informed by a theoretical framework.

The assessment requires the ability to stay with a difficult subject for some time and not be diverted into talking about something more comfortable. If the family appears uncomfortable with a certain line of questioning, then the practitioner needs to draw on his or her skills to gently reframe their questions. It is crucial that the parent or child does not feel 'judged' and feels sufficiently secure at least to reflect on the issues being raised. A training manual supported by the Department of Health – *The Family Assessment: Assessment of Family Competence, Strengths, and Difficulties* – is an excellent resource for practitioners seeking further guidance on how to complete a systemic assessment (Bentovim and Bingley Miller 2001).

Method of assessment

The assessment needs to consider the child within his or her *family system*. Secondly, it aims to consider the impact of the death on the wider *community system* – for example, school, friends, religious institution, sports clubs, and so on – and thirdly it assesses the *situational factors* arising from the death itself: for example, if the death was by suicide. Much of the information-gathering begins through drawing up a genogram.

Genograms have several functions in a bereavement assessment:

- On a purely practical level genograms provide a written account of *who is who* in the family.

- Genograms help to identify *previous losses* – and to gauge their severity based on the perceptions of family members.

- Genograms also allow the practitioner to identify how the family has *coped with such previous losses.* They can explore which coping strategies were positive and helpful, and identify potential trends that proved unhelpful. For example, a parent might say: 'When I lost my job I suppose I turned to drinking quite heavily' and, in response, questions such as: 'Have you found yourself drinking more since Marion's death?' may be legitimately explored.

- Finally, the genogram can be used to determine the impact of the death on the *current family system.* In particular, are there any *key transitions* for this family, such as moving schools, marital separations, emigrations, weddings, retirements, serious illness in another family member, conflict relationships, dependency issues, or other current or imminent issues?

Throughout the general assessment process, the practitioner needs to be mindful of the factors which may have promoted *resilience* throughout childhood (Stokes 2009) (see Table 5.1). Shuurman (2003) developed a comparison of bereaved children and resilient children (see Table 5.2). Shuurman believes: 'the key at-risk factor bereaved children demonstrate in greater proportion than their non-bereaved peers is an external locus of control. Resilient children have a strong belief that they can control their fates by their own actions; bereaved children show a higher evidence of externalizing control, believing that their fate is in someone else's hands'. (Shuurman 2003).

Table 5.1 Assessing resilience in childhood

- Strong social support networks
- The presence of at least one unconditionally supportive parent or parent substitute
- Positive school experiences
- A sense of mastery and a belief that one's own efforts can make a difference
- Participation in events outside school and the home
- The capacity to reframe adversities so that the beneficial effects are recognized
- The ability – or the opportunity – to make a difference by helping others or through part-time work (for teenagers)
- Not to be excessively sheltered from challenging situations which provide opportunities to develop coping skills

---

Source: (Newman 2002)

Table 5.2

The significant seven characteristics of bereaved children	Five personality traits or predispositions of resilient children
External locus of control	Internal locus of control
Lower self-esteem	Healthy self-esteem
Higher levels of anxiety/fearfulness	Easy-going temperament
Higher evidence of depression	Affectionate
More accidents and health problems	Good reasoning skills
Pessimism about the future	
Under performing	

Source: (Schuurman 2003)

Before the assessment

Research consistently shows that it is not easy for parents to connect emotionally to their children's grief (Dyregrov 1991). However, the literature also concludes that parents often have the greatest influence on their child's adjustment (Silverman 2000). It is therefore crucial to engage the parent or carer, and for them to feel confident with the assessment process. It can be helpful to telephone a parent before a home visit to check if there are any issues they are concerned about discussing in front of the children. This can liberate a parent reluctant to access services because they feel paralyzed by a 'secret', for example: 'I can't face telling the children that their brother killed himself ... not yet anyway'. In time, we would usually hope to work towards a family understanding of the suicide – however, it is very important that the parent feels in control of the information-sharing process. It is not the role of a child bereavement service to 'take over' and enforce principles of open, honest discussion before the time feels right for the parent.

The importance of engaging the whole family

Parents may need to keep their children home from school so that the whole family gets the most out of the assessment. As the school will need an explanation for absence this can provide an opportunity to reinforce the school's awareness that a child in its care is coping with a significant bereavement. In family discussions when the children are present, practitioners need to take care to use words that children can understand so that they do not feel excluded.

The home setting

Assessments which take place in a family's home will need to follow policy guidelines addressing the health and safety issues involved in home visiting.

When it is time for the children to be interviewed, the practitioners ask them where they would like to talk. This is often their bedroom, or a separate room downstairs. Parental consent must be given for any room used. Doors should be left open and child protection guidelines followed.

Absent family members

Practitioners also need to plan how they will respond if key family members are missing. There is a balance between affirming and working with those who attend while explaining how difficult it is to get to know the family as a whole without the presence and perspective of key members. Asking a family's views about how the absent member(s) might respond to a further invitation to attend can be a good way of exploring family realities (Bentovim and Bingley Miller 2001, Stokes et al. 2009).

Family members who are reluctant to join in

Sometimes a parent might say: 'Simon is home, but he is in his room and doesn't want to come down'. In such situations it can be useful to ask who in the family would be best at persuading the child to come in, and perhaps sending them to see the child with a message from you. The approach could be something like this: 'Am I right in thinking Simon is upstairs and not sure about joining us? Could someone in the family go and say from me that it would be great if he could join us, even for a short while? Who would be best to do that?'

Framework for a home assessment

Although each home assessment is tailored to meet each individual family's needs, the visit is likely to take place flexibly within the following framework.

Understanding the reason for the visit

With all the family together, the practitioners will need to check that the child(ren) know about the reason for the visit.

Rationale for assessment

It is necessary to ensure that the child(ren) understand that the visit is not because they have been naughty or are 'sick' but that it is quite natural and usual to help when an important person in someone's life has died.

Referrer

If the parent was not the referrer then it may be appropriate to talk about the person who made contact, and their connections with the family.

Explaining the assessment format

Starting on time, and continuing to keep to the agreed time boundaries, is one indication to the family that you will work professionally and respectfully with them. In explaining the format for the visit the practitioner could suggest for a family with a mother and two children (called John and Vicky): 'What we would like to do now is suggest that perhaps I have a chance to talk with mum on her own. John, perhaps you could meet with my colleague Jim? That means that Vicky can have a break for half an hour until John and Jim have finished. Does that sound OK? When we've finished we will all catch up together as a family and we can talk about the ways we may be able to help'.

Establishing rapport

When making an assessment of the emotional, cognitive, and behavioural issues arising from the death, the practitioner will explain *why* it is necessary to explore these avenues. The parent or child needs to feel *in control* of what information they choose to share. For example, asking about 'your partner' rather than 'your husband' might make it easier to explain that a couple were not married or that their partner was the same sex.

Utilizing a family tree to gather information

As mentioned previously, a useful way to begin the assessment is to construct a family tree or *genogram*. Children often enjoy doing this, and it can give the practitioner valuable insights into how the family functions. For example, it becomes clear how much the children know about their family, how the parent(s) and children communicate with each other, and the level of respect each shows for the other in the way they give and share information.

It is usually helpful to have different colours or symbols for male and female, for people who are alive and those who have died and so on. It is also useful to put dates on for deaths and separations, including divorces. The practitioner may want to invite the family to show, again through symbols or colours, who is especially close or has particularly distant or ambivalent relationships. The discussion can focus on a range of aspects using these techniques. Finding out what influence the family perceives other members from past generations have had on them can provide useful and interesting information. Asking who takes after whom can help to identify ways in which the family members are bringing forward their understanding of the past.

However, it is likely that the parent will, at times, decide to protect the children from certain information. If the genogram is completed with the children present, the practitioner will need to check out later if there was anything that the parent had chosen not to mention in front of the children. A parent might then say, for example: 'I didn't like to mention this in front of Becky, but my husband was actually married before and so Becky has a half sister'.

In constructing a genogram the practitioner will also try to establish family members' own perspective of themselves and to see how far they recognize their strengths and difficulties. This can provide a useful insight into the resilience demonstrated by the family as a whole. It also gives an indication of the degree to which the relationships in the family are supportive and appreciative, or otherwise, and how the family attributes strengths and difficulties. 'Even though dad has died we are still a family'.

The following case study provides an overview of the process outlined in constructing a genogram. In particular, it is intended to show careful cross-referencing, establishing the 'meaning' which each family member gives to the 'facts' as they emerge.

By constructing a genogram (see Fig. 5.1), the practitioner would quickly identify a number of key facts and issues, a few of which are listed overleaf. Taken in isolation these facts tell us very little: the richness comes when the *meaning and relevance of these issues to various family members* have been discussed in order to complete the picture of interwoven threads.

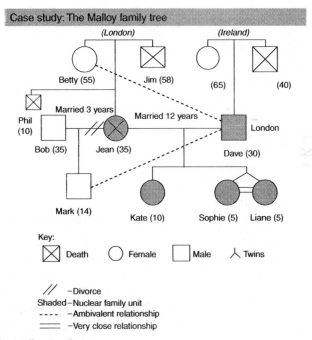

Fig. 5.1 The Malloy Family tree.

The following information was obtained when drawing the genogram with the children's father (Dave):

- Dave and Jean had been married for 12 years and they had three daughters. Jean had been married before: the marriage lasted three years and she had a son (Mark) from the marriage who is now 14.

- Jean died in a road traffic accident. She was not driving; the driver survived. Jean was not wearing a seatbelt. She was 35 years old.

- Kate was a passenger and witnessed her mother's death. She is showing symptoms of post-traumatic stress.

- Kate is in her last year at primary school. She will change to a secondary school in September.

- Dave is currently thinking that this might be a good time to make a fresh start by moving closer to his mother who lives in Ireland.

- Dave's father died suddenly aged 40. Dave was 8 at the time, and he will be 40 next year.

- Mark, a stepbrother, has a volatile relationship with his stepdad (Dave) which worsened significantly when his mother died.

- After Jean's death Mark decided to move back to live with his father. He is still local and hasn't changed school.

- Sophie and Liane are together in the reception year at school. Jean had decided with the school that the twins would go into separate classes after completion of their reception year.

- Dave has a complicated relationship with Jean's mother, who has expressed her belief that he is 'too busy' with his job to care properly for the children. She helps with household chores and insists that all Jean's things remain in place.

- Betty is devastated by her daughter's death but seems hard to reach and needs to blame others.

- Betty is in close contact with Mark.

- Betty's husband (Jean's father) died last year. The cause of death was confirmed as suicide, from carbon monoxide poisoning in a car. Jim had struggled with depression since his son's death from leukaemia 20 years earlier. He died on his son's birthday.

- The children were told that their grandfather had had an accident in the car. Dave said he felt uncomfortable with this explanation as it was misleading.

- Bob (Jean's first husband) enjoyed a good relationship with both Jean and Dave. 'They married young, had Mark, but split up when he was a baby'. Bob lives close by and tries to build bridges between Mark and Dave.

These are just *some* of the many issues which emerged, helping the practitioner to build a picture of the impact of Jean's death, at this particular time, for this particular family, living in this particular community.

The smaller picture

Understanding different viewpoints – illustrated by taking one specific issue arising from this assessment

The practitioner's role is to establish facts and then try to understand their meaning for different family members. *It is not just the actual facts themselves which determine risk – it is the meaning that different family members give to them.* Using an example from this genogram we could reflect on the meaning different people might have for the seemingly inconsequential plan to separate the twins when they return for their second year at school. While this had been agreed with Jean, as part of the school's policy, the plan took on a different meaning for different people after her death.

Dave's view

Since Jean's death Dave is desperate to make sure that the family feels safe and secure. He says Jean was really good at this and he sometimes feels he doesn't know where to start. He is anxious that nothing unnecessary should upset the balance of family life. Dave remembers a long period of refusing to go to school when his father died. His mother was happy for him to stay at home and responded protectively to even fairly minor physical symptoms. Dave is worried that the girls are starting to do the same, and he knows this will be difficult with his work. 'I just want to do my best for the girls. At times I feel like running away because it's all too much. The twins being put into separate classes is the final straw!' Dave says that he feels furious with the school and strongly believes that regular stomach aches experienced by the twins are connected to their worries about being separated from him and each other.

Sophie's view

Sophie seems to have become more dependent on Liane; she is unusually aggressive. Sophie says she is scared that boys at school will make jokes about the fact that her mum has died. 'I want to be with my sister, always'.

Liane's view

The quieter twin, she frequently wets herself at school and is rarely vocal, allowing her sister to speak on her behalf. Liane whispered to the practitioner: 'I wish my dad could give up work so I can stay at home, or perhaps mum can come back from heaven'.

The school's view

With Dave's permission, the school was telephoned after the home assessment. The head teacher explained that he has not yet personally spoken to Dave about the twins. 'Dave has got so much on his plate that I don't want to burden him further at the moment. I'd be happy to talk about next year when he is ready'. The girls' class teacher believes that Liane would benefit from greater independence from Sophie, but is reluctant to say this to Dave as she senses his vulnerability and quick temper. So, it would appear that a breakdown in communication has meant that Dave now perceives the school as being cold and inflexible, and gives him further evidence for his belief that he is isolated and vulnerable.

So, it is only after the practitioner has gleaned an understanding from various perspectives that they can then try to generate a hypothesis about what is going on and how a seemingly small issue, such as the twins' school attendance, needs to be moved forward or resolved in a positive way while the family is in crisis.

The bigger picture

Assessing risk and resilience

The overall assessment revealed a variety of issues which informed the practitioners how past family history affects and how different family members are coping with Jean's death. In addition, it identified the impact of her death having occurred at this particular time: for example, Kate will soon be changing to secondary school, Dave is considering moving to Ireland, the twins had just started school and it is only a year since the maternal grandfather died by suicide. Family members hold differing views on the factors which led to both the grandfather's and Jean's deaths.

The assessment process aims to unravel how different family members reacted to previous losses and, again, to relate this to the current situation. For example, while Dave was understanding about Betty's devastation following the deaths of her children and husband, he felt frustrated by her emotional outbursts and angry that she couldn't offer more practical help with child care. He also felt that Betty intensified the difficulties he had in relating to Mark.

While the assessment is about collecting information, it can also become an intervention in itself especially if the practitioner uses techniques (such as circular questioning) to loosen family assumptions. For example, questions such as 'Who do you think is most upset about mum's death? If I asked dad if he was thinking of moving to Ireland what do you think he would say? If granny Betty could have three wishes what do you think they would be? If you could have three wishes what would you ask for? If I had met your family before mum died, what would an average week have been like?' could be asked. At the end of 2–3 hours the assessment was completed. The family reported feeling both exhausted but relieved to have spoken so openly and honestly.

Sharing information with the rest of the family

The family regroups once all the individual interviews have taken place. It is important for everyone to check out what information they are willing to have shared when the family unit 'regroups'. Sometimes the practitioners will need to reframe ideas for the children: this may enable the children to share something in a way that they believe will be more acceptable to their parent. For example, the practitioner might say: 'You know you said that your mum is always shouting and angry since your dad died … when we meet back up with mum would it be OK to say something like: "The children have noticed that you sometimes seem to be more irritable and tired since their dad died, and they were wondering if they could help in any way?"'

Closing the assessment and leaving the family with a task

If appropriate, families are introduced to the possibility of choosing or developing their own memory box. The rationale is explained, and children and parents are invited to share ideas on how they might build up the contents of their own individual box. This exercise provides a stimulating closing activity for the assessment and, in addition, leaves a tangible attachment and reminder of the purpose of meeting with the family.

Planning appropriate interventions

Before leaving, the practitioner will give a broad outline of what they think might be the best way forward. In terms of the programme available at Winston's Wish this could be a combination of some of the following:

(a) Family invited to attend a residential weekend group (25 children)

(b) Group intervention offered when the cause of death is (i) murder/manslaughter; (ii) suicide

(c) In situations where the assessment has identified trauma or complicated grief, individual work may be offered to a parent and/or a child

(d) Teenagers may prefer to attend an outward bound weekend specifically for 14-18 year olds. (No parental involvement, unlike the other residential weekends above)

(e) Children under 5 may be invited to attend a weekly 6 session group with their parents

(f) Agreement to discuss the assessment with external agencies, most importantly the child's teacher

(g) Referral on to another agency for issues identified during the assessment and outside the aims of the Winston's Wish programme e.g. welfare/financial assistance, severe eating disorder, etc

(h) The family specifically request no further contact.

This chapter has explored the ways in which a detailed assessment can guide the most appropriate intervention for each family. Assessment of family functioning, and of the wider context in which a child exists, is one of the hardest yet most important skills a practitioner has to develop. The well-being of bereaved children depends on our being able to identify those strengths within a family on which we can build, and to define those difficulties we are aiming to help alleviate. The assessment can be viewed as an intricate dance, where the practitioner may well know the 'steps' but has the confidence to allow the 'rhythm' to be determined by the family.

References

Bentovim, A. Bingley Miller, L. (2001) *The Family Assessment: Assessment of Family competence, strengths, and Difficulties*. Brighton: Pavilion Publishing.

Dyregrov, A. (1991) *Grief in children: A handbook for adults*. London: Jessica Kingsley.

Glaser, D., Furniss, T., and Bingley, L. (1984) Focal Family Therapy: The Assessment Stage. *Journal of Family Therapy*, **4**: 132–77.

Greenhalgh, T. (2002) Uneasy bedfellows? Reconciling intuition and evidence-based practice. *Young Minds Magazine*, **59**: 23–7.

Newman, T. (2002) *Promoting Resilience: A Review of Effective Strategies for Child Care Services*. University of Exeter: Centre for Evidence Based Social Sciences: www.exeter.ac.uk/cebss

Parkes, C.M., and Weiss, R.S. (1983) *Recovery from Bereavement*. New York: Basic Books, pp. 31–4.

Schuurman, D. (2003) *Never the Same – Coming to Terms With the Death of a Parent*. New York: St Martin's Press, pp. 130–1.

Shapiro, E.R. (1994) *Grief as a Family Process: A Developmental Approach to Clinical Practice*. New York: Guilford Press.

Silverman, P.R. (2000) *Never Too Young to Know: Death in Children's Lives*. New York: Oxford University Press.

Stokes, J. (2009). Resilience and Bereaved Children – Helping a child to develop a resilient mindset following the death of a parent. *Bereavement Care*. **28**(1). Routledge.

Stokes, J. Cook, V. and Reed, C. (2009) Life as an adolescent when a parent has died. In Balk, D.C., and Corr, C.A. (eds). *Adolescent Encounters with Death, Bereavement and Coping*. New York: Springer.

Stubbs, D. Ailovick, K. Stokes, J. Howells, K. (2006) *Family Asssessment: Guidelines for Child Bereavement Practitioners*. Cheltenham, UK: Winston's Wish.

Chapter 6

Therapeutic interventions

Patsy Way and Isobel Bremner

Introduction

We are members of the Candle Project team at St Christopher's Hospice. Isobel comes from a psychodynamic background and Patsy works from a systemic family therapy tradition. Our methods are similar in that we offer a brief intervention to children and families, usually with a maximum of six sessions in child-friendly surroundings in St Christopher's Hospice in South London. We have a playroom with art, craft, and play materials and a slightly larger room, suitable for older teenagers and families.

In this chapter we outline our thinking in making specific interventions with a particular child, young person, or family. For convenience, Patsy begins by reflecting on the family perspective and discusses techniques with children and families, and Isobel then describes work with adolescents, though we both work with both groups. Names and identifying features of children and young people we work with have been changed to protect confidentiality.

The family perspective

Context of work

Our primary brief in the Candle Project is to support bereaved children and young people but this must inevitably involve their families. Parent/carers are our co-partners in this task, bringing their knowledge and concerns about their children following a bereavement while we bring a particular expertise in thinking and talking about some difficult areas around death and bereavement. In south London we meet a wide variety of cultures, ethnicities and religious traditions, but all families are unique and have developed their own complex culture.

The context for bereavement work with children varies greatly in different projects; at the Candle Project we meet children and families in our own setting and do no home visits. In a small team, we are able to offer up to six sessions and will meet the parent/carer first. This in itself can be a very therapeutic intervention, though the primary focus is on the children in the family. Very occasionally a young person has been unwilling for us to discuss their issues with parents and, in this situation, we have referred on to a teenage counselling service with a different brief on teenagers and confidentiality.

Team members may liaise with parent/carers in different ways. Some meet a child or young person and then feed back parts of the conversation to the parent/carer, with the child/young person's agreement. Sometimes some or all members of the family are included in a meeting, and there may be variations in who is involved in different sessions. Clarity about the limits of confidentiality and the organizational stance on children's safety are important, and children and adults need to understand what will be shared with others in the family.

Referral

Referrals may come from the family or other networks, such as the family doctor or the school, who will also have a perspective on events surrounding the bereavement. Quite often some form of behaviour on the part of the child or young person has prompted a referral. A child may appear to the referrer to be too distressed or not showing enough emotion. They may be seen to be showing a lot of anger towards others or turning inwards and hurting themselves. At a time when all family members are deeply distressed following bereavement and carers struggle with managing the immediate practical demands of the situation, it may be very difficult for family members to see the child's response as connected to their own.

Bereaved children do not have the power to change their immediate circumstances, and sometimes the family is swept on a tide of changes and additional stressors with barely time for explanation to a child about what is happening. A child behaving angrily may be seen as exerting immense destructive power in the family in ways perceived as negative, aggressive and violent.

Case study

Ryan, aged 8, came into the room with eyes lowered, followed by his mother and two sisters. When I asked why the children thought they were here they all looked at Ryan and he announced (still without looking at me) that it was because he was 'being bad' since dad died.

I asked how I would know if different members of the family were feeling cross, and I showed some cartoons demonstrating 'styles' of anger. His younger sister admitted that when she felt angry she sometimes provoked others and then complained she was a target. His older sister admitted to sometimes clowning around to distract and deflect her anger. His mother agreed that she was shouting at the children much more since her husband's death. We developed the idea that everyone has different ways of showing anger. Some anger styles are more effective and useful than others, but we sometimes get stuck and default to a particular way of showing our rage. In talking about when and how they got angry the family moved into discussions around how these feelings might connect to sad ones, following their father's death. Ryan's mother Maryanne pointed out proudly that Ryan had been very 'strong' and not cried and later said that she worried that Ryan showed so little emotion at the funeral.

I pulled out my box of 'feelings balls' and invited them to connect a feeling to each ball. There emerged a pink one for happy feelings, one with a plastic shark inside for scary feelings, an uneven one for confusion, a blue one for sadness, and a bright red one for angry feelings. I asked who would be most likely to catch the angry ball in the family. Everyone agreed this was Ryan and the ball was thrown to him. However, different examples were given of how the others also showed their anger, and the ball started to travel round the room with his sisters and mother accepting it and describing ways they showed their anger. Soon the anger and sadness balls were being thrown together as connections were made.

The 'homework' following this session was for each person to notice their own 'style' of feeling upset, and when and where this was most likely to show. During the next session they all contributed to the discussion about how the bereavement had affected them and the focus was no longer solely on Ryan and his 'bad behaviour'.

Bereavement as a transition

Whether sudden or after a long illness, families often face a time of confusion as they negotiate changes of roles and position in the family after bereavement. The future is not what was expected. During a transitional period, everyone is uncertain about how to behave and act into a new situation. If someone died or left a position in an organization there would be recognized, formal ways of managing the transition. The post would be advertised with job and person specifications. In a family context there is rarely such clarity about roles. In the midst of adult distress and confusion, communication often becomes more fraught and children, who may have the least understanding, are often afforded the least information. Sometimes their concerns can seem trivial to adults, as when Sarah's father had just died in a tragic car crash and she demanded, 'But who is going to take me to school?' Behind the question lay all the uncertainties that follow the loss of a key member of the family. Children can keenly feel family tensions and be very aware of how they might be repositioned after a death, for example in the case of an eldest boy following the death of a father. Worden (1996 p14) suggests the need for paying 'particular attention to feelings of ambivalence and responsibility'.

Walsh and McGoldrick (1995 pp7-13) echo Worden's (1991) four tasks of mourning but frame the tasks in a family context suggesting that, following bereavement, the family has the adaptational tasks of:

- acknowledging together the reality of the death and experiencing the loss
- reorganizing the family system and reinvesting in other relationships and life pursuits.

Such tasks may make great demands on communication patterns in the family. Children may mirror coping and communication styles demonstrated by family members (Worden 1996) who themselves may be oscillating confusingly between loss and restoration behaviours (Stroebe and Schut 1999). If there are tensions in coping styles, children sometimes either accommodate to adults, perhaps by restraining their own expressions of emotion, or distract, as in situations where a focus on a child's behaviour in school may deflect from the enormity of the grief. Communication can become very complex where different family members have only partial information, as for example about a suicide (Dyregrov and Dyregrov 2008).

Most grief theories, developing through ideas of attachment and loss, have focused on individuals, with little attention to relational aspects of bereavement. However, from a constructivist position, Neimeyer (2001) has discussed the familial and cultural factors that shape our efforts after meaning, arguing that families need support in reconstructing their story to enable them to make coherent sense of their past, present, and futures as they become a different kind of family after the death.

Based on her research, Nadeau (1998) emphasized the ways in which family members interact to construct meanings around a death and adds to our understanding of grief theory by showing the wide range of meanings made in families and the processes involved, demonstrating how family dynamics, structure, ways of talking and contextual features impact on outcomes in bereavement.

Despite the challenges, Christ's research (2000 p242) validates the strengths of families and affirms that, 'Surviving parents can grieve deeply but can still be available to their children' and children can move forward in developmentally appropriate ways. Stokes (2007) notes key family factors that impact positively on the resilience of a bereaved child including: a stable and supportive home environment, a warm parenting style offering clear boundaries, and the interest and involvement of the parent in education. Important also is the parent/carer's willingness to accept support for the family.

Techniques for working with bereaved children

The techniques outlined below draw on a range of thinking, notably the work of Wilson (1998) and Freeman et al. (1997) in promoting very playful approaches with families that create an atmosphere in which children and adults feel comfortable in tackling serious issues with a minimal sense of being blamed.

Burnham (1992) has made a distinction between approach, method, and technique in a piece of work, noting that counsellors might share similar approaches but have very different methods and techniques or perhaps, as in this case, come from different approaches but have similarities on methods and/or techniques. The focus here is on techniques.

Why use play? Different techniques for different purposes

When first meeting a parent/carer or family I ask why they have chosen to access the Candle Project at this point in bereavement and what they are hoping for. It is crucial that the intervention and the focus of the work is clearly defined and that the techniques chosen for work with a family can engage the imagination and creative energies of both children and adults together (Lewis and Kavanagh 1995). Playful techniques are used as a language to connect with children. These ideas are intended not as prescriptions for intervention but more as a stimulus for creative responses to engage children.

Learning about the family: getting started

Engaging parent/carers and children in drawing a family tree together can provide a way into understanding how members of a family tell stories about themselves and their deceased relatives and also what understanding children have about events surrounding the bereavement.

Case study

Mrs F came with four children under seven years old. Their grandfather, a native of Ghana, who had lived in the family home, had been murdered. He had been a very significant figure for the children as their father no longer had contact. I invited Mrs F and each child to choose a different coloured felt tip to draw up a family tree with me. Explaining that we use a circle for a girl or woman and square for boy or man, I invited children to write their names and ages. As family, friends, and pets were added to the tree in turn, children and adults elaborated on how they played a role in their lives, telling anecdotes about an aunt, her cat, her favourite food, what happened when …. All this enabled a conversation that included even the youngest in the room, allowed the children a growing confidence in working with me and gave me a view on how this family communicate together, who takes the lead, who is most listened to, and what is acceptable to say or not say.

One of the twins hesitated about drawing in his goldfish, who had died, on the family tree. The six year old used the phrase 'Lost my grandad' and was unsure where his grandfather was lost. On the way to heaven? In Ghana? This allowed opportunities to unfold the story of how grandad died, what happened to his body (including explanations that his body couldn't see, feel or talk), the body being sent back to Ghana, and the burial. We were able to look up Ghana on the map and see it was a long way away but a real place, a place the children might visit one day. We talked about funerals (using picture books) and what happens and what people do. We talked about heaven (this is a churchgoing family) as a different kind of place. We discussed differences between body and spirit. I was given openings for conversations in future sessions with the older girls, who were left with issues of anger, guilt, forgiveness, and retribution.

The drawing up of family maps or family trees allows a professional a way into conversations, and an opportunity to understand more of how this family works together.

Checking in: what else is happening in your life (Including the good things!)

When someone dies children's worlds may be turned upside down with a series of secondary losses. Some families will have economic stressors after a family member dies. The remaining parent/carer may be taking a new job and the family may need to move. Children may be looked after differently, families split, and young people may need to change schools. Children and families may not be recognizing the effect of this on themselves and the way they connect with each other. I developed a 'how's it going?' sheet to address these areas. This can be done quickly and non-verbally at the beginning of sessions. It allows me an insight into how the child/ren experienced the intervening time since the last meeting. It allows children to tell me more about areas I might not know or ask about, or that they might think irrelevant to bereavement. Five categories address health, relationships with adults in school, parent/carers and peers and a general 'feelings' section. The child is invited to tick the illustration best reflecting their recent experience. If parent/carers or others in the family are present they can comment from their point of view. Children can then decide whether to tell me more about, for example, an upsetting episode at home, or keep it private. The sheet can be completed very quickly and put aside or become the basis of the whole session if interesting and important stories emerge.

Case study

Sam is nine years old and without siblings. He has been trying so hard to be helpful to his mother Jane, who talks about him as 'my little man', helping with cooking, washing up, and locking up the house at night as his father used to. He is confused and uncertain about his father's death six months ago, when he fell on a railway line following an alcoholic binge. The school has tried hard not to worry Jane who they see as distraught and finding it hard to be available to her son. Another child taunted him in the playground with, 'Where's your dad then?' On using the check in sheet Sam said, 'it's not really about dad but ...' and recounted the story of how he had reacted by fighting because he felt upset and confused, not knowing the answer to the question. I asked questions about what he could ask his mother. Jane in turn gave voice to her love and concern for Sam in spite of her sadness. We could then think about practical strategies for managing such incidents in school, inviting the support of his class teacher.

In a subsequent session we addressed Sam's wider worries, inviting him to draw a cross-section of his brain, showing the proportion of his thinking taken up with different things.

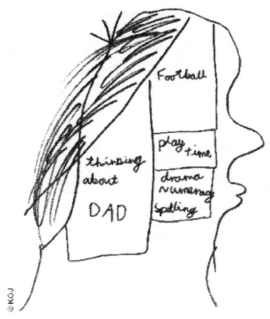

Fig. 6.1 Brain cross-section: Sam's brain.

Case study

Jane was amazed at how much of his attention he showed as thoughts of his dad and worries about her health and abilities to cope. She had imagined he was rather irritatingly absent at times and showing general laziness and inattention in school. This image started a conversation that led onto discussions about what each could expect from the other. It allowed for explanations and reassurances that, although she was stressed and unhappy, she was not terminally ill as he feared. We explored Sam's questions about 'dad on the railway' and Jane explained in simple language about the coroner having found out all about it, like a detective, and deciding that his father had fallen under the train, probably because his brain was all muddled up from drinking the beer, but that we do not know exactly what happened or why. Sam asked if his father might have done it on purpose and Jane said this was possible but she did not know. She reassured him that she and his father loved him very much and if his father had made that kind of mistake when his head was muddled from the drink, it was not to do with Sam because his father and she loved him very much.

Externalizing

We know (Rowling 2003) that 'gender can be a significant disenfranchising issue for young males in schools' and that bereaved boys are more likely to show behaviours in school likely to lead to serious consequences and sometimes permanent exclusion. Bereaved children are often managing a series of secondary losses which may impact on their lives for a long time. Boys often react with anger and aggression when confused and upset, which then attracts an angry response. White (1990) developed ideas of 'externalising' some behaviours as a technique for shifting the blame outside of the individual, particularly when one member of the family appears to carry the weight of criticism.

Case study

Junior is six years old. His teacher complains that, though she knows he is a bright boy, he behaves differently since his older brother died. His brother had special needs and suffered from a complex medical condition. Though there had always been concerns about his disabilities there had not been any expectation that he would die so young and suddenly. Junior's teacher, though initially very sympathetic, feels that more than a year after the death this can no longer be an excuse for Junior's isolated and angry behaviours in school, which are causing him to lose friends and his teachers to lose patience. Junior's mother, bereaved and utterly exhausted, is exasperated. At home Junior is generally helpful and caring towards her with only occasional outbursts of temper. She is attending frequent meetings in school about what is described as his increasingly aggressive and antisocial behaviour. She would agree with his teachers that bereavement can no longer be an excuse.

I began asking whether Junior was familiar with Roger Hargreaves' books about the 'Mr Men'. His favourite was Mr Tickle and, following a conversation with him and his mother about events in school, I wondered aloud if 'Mr Angry' might have been visiting him. Would he be more likely to visit him at home or at school? In the classroom or in the playground? When his teacher was there or not? Did he visit anyone else at home or at school? Junior pointed out that there wasn't really a Mr Angry and I replied, inviting him into a playful and imaginative space, saying, 'How would we know? Perhaps there is?'

Junior looked intrigued and I expanded my theme that perhaps Mr Angry might be sneaking up to him when he was most vulnerable in the classroom and inviting him to the kicking, punching and rude behaviours that upset his classmates and teachers.

I wondered what Mr Angry might look like and Junior began to create him out of playdough using a kit that provides little plastic arms, legs, eyes and hats while I chatted to him, asking about how Mr Angry might be affecting his life. Junior engaged playfully, answering questions such as, 'If he invites you to do these things, what are the consequences?' It got Junior himself into big trouble, upset his mother, teachers and school friends and the only person who would enjoy it all would be Mr Angry himself. I wondered aloud if Mr Angry might not have a team of nasty characters egging him on, such as Mr Punch, Mr Temper, and Mr Not-Pay-Attention.

Junior made them all in turn in playdough and as he did so, I asked him for more detail about how these characters were spoiling his life in school. I pointed out that we, of course, knew that this was not the 'real' Junior, who, from previous descriptions, was very helpful and supportive of his mother. I began to wonder about a team of other characters, led by Mr Helpful, who invited Junior to behaviours that others enjoyed and admired. Finally I set Junior and his mother some 'homework'. We took a Polaroid photo of him with the playdough characters, to be put on the fridge door. Junior and his mother were to note down any time when they thought Mr Angry and friends were going to invite Junior into unhelpful behaviours but he managed to listen to Mr Helpful and his crew.

At the next meeting, Junior's mother reported on times she had noticed James escaping from Mr Angry, some occasions that Junior himself had not noticed until pointed out. Junior enjoyed explaining to me in detail how he had, with support from Mr Helpful, chosen to act differently in school also. His mother had taken a friendly classroom assistant, Mrs Jones, into their confidence and she was also alert to 'escapes' from Mr Angry and company in the school playground and relayed these observations to the class teacher. I could then offer certificates and stickers to recognize these important escapes. This also enabled a conversation about when and how anger can be useful and necessary and I could then invite Junior to think about how he experienced anger in his body, and how he chose to deal with it and manage it in different situations at home and school.

In this externalizing technique White invites children to look at their behavioural choices from a position of not feeling blamed, on the premise that change is more likely to occur when one is not defending one's behaviour. Externalising allows other, forgotten, and more positive descriptions of a child to re-emerge, and allows all those involved to separate the behaviours from the person.

Case study

In the final session, Junior drew Mr Angry and we photocopied him in different sizes. Junior thought Mr Angry was now 'pocket sized' and manageable and might have some uses. As he got bigger, however, he was not helpful, so that an A3 sized Mr Angry would probably cause more trouble for him in school. The classroom assistant and his mother were then able to ask Junior how big Mr Angry was on a particular day, and take their cue on how much nurturing and monitoring Junior was asking for. This enabled a supportive dialogue to begin to develop between home and school, no longer focusing on blaming Junior.

Ways of remembering

Some techniques are well described in the literature. For example, Winston's Wish in their 'Muddles, Puddles and Sunshine' activity book (2000) describe use of a memory box for treasures which relate to or belonged to the deceased. Similarly, I describe below my use of memory jars (Stokes 2004 p78) to enrich a child's narrative of precious memories of a dead person. Memory jars are one of many ways of using colour association to talk with a child about special memories.

Case study

Jenny's mother, Wendy, died nearly a year ago. Jenny is an only child and, like her father, is struggling to weave memories of Wendy into a new life without her. We made a memory jar using a recycled spice jar and salt coloured with chalks.

Jenny put blue salt in the first layer of the jar, reminding her of a visit to the sea, before her mother was wheelchair bound. A layer of pink salt followed, evoking the pink icing on the birthday cake her mother had ordered specially for her fifth birthday, and mauve reminded her of Wendy's nightgown when she was ill and Jenny visited her in hospital. A range of similar colour association techniques can be used such as marbling kits. Coloured inks require no artistic talent to use and always result in interesting and pleasing swirls of colour.

Time line: a connecting narrative between past, present, and future

Michael White (1989) invites the bereaved to 'say hello again' to the deceased. Having mourned the loss and changes in their lives he suggests ways of working with people to bring that person into their present and future thinking. This has resonances with Tony Walter's work (1999) and Continuing Bonds (Klass et al. 1996). Children and families are sometimes uncertain of how someone who has been central in their lives can continue to be part of their present and future as well as being held in past memory. Many are afraid of memories fading and feeling that the person will then be lost forever. I have adapted ideas from White (2001) which I have presented here as a time line.

Case study

Laura is 11 and about to transfer to secondary school, losing the familiarity of a small primary setting where everyone knows her. She is the eldest of three girls and her mother died of cancer eight months ago after a long illness which began after the birth of the youngest child. Laura has been 'the little mother' during two house moves, illness and remissions. Her father, who is attentive and concerned about her, has a new partner who is pregnant. Laura herself has just had her first period. In the next few months Laura will have a new sibling, a new caring adult, and a new school. Recently she has been bad tempered and uncharacteristically aggressive. She is usually seen as friendly, helpful and competent, appreciated by family, friends, and teachers.

In our meeting, I pulled out a roll of wallpaper and we drew two parallel lines. The bottom one was the time line on which we recorded important dates and events, from her parents' first meeting and her birth and continuing on into her future and adulthood. I asked her and her father about the qualities they valued in her and how she had developed these.

Stories emerged of patience and competence in looking after babies and her ill mother. They spoke of her drama skills in school, encouraged by her mother, her funny jokes and dances as a little girl. She was described attending to her mother's needs for gentleness, quiet and distraction at different stages of the illness.

We connected this (literally, with a coloured felt-tip) to events and stories that included other family members and friends, noticing how she was the same and also different from her mother. A rich story emerged of Laura's developing skills and qualities over time, nurtured by her mother and others. We projected these into the future and I asked questions such as, 'I wonder how these abilities will show in your new school? How will this ability to connect and communicate with others develop in college or university? In your first job? With your first boyfriend?'

In this way particular memories were deepened, and in the process of telling and listening to these memories, descriptions of Laura that connected her with her mother and others and emphasized her strengths and resourcefulness were linked with her past, present and future. This allowed new conversations to develop around her place in her newly forming family, and the way in which Laura and her abilities are valued. This included her father's new partner and the baby in her present and future, and allowed her to talk about her mother with them in a way that did not invite her to feel disloyal to her memory or to new and emerging aspects of her own identity.

The last session

The last session provides an opportunity to review the work and think about changes that have happened and are hoped for, including the deceased in thinking about the past, present and future and perhaps putting together a little book of the worksheets. Ending rituals of photographs and the gift of a little bear mark the parting and an 'extended warranty' is offered and a child will be invited to a group. Parents may also be encouraged to attend a group.

Techniques for working with bereaved young people

Bereaved young people are managing the turbulence of both adolescence and grief. They will be experiencing the pressure of secondary education, a growing awareness of sexual feelings, and significant changes in their bodies, and a drive towards separating from their parents/carers. They have probably not explicitly asked for help with their bereavement and may feel aggrieved that anyone would think that they need support from a professional. This is the context in which much work with young people begins, so how do we make a connection and move forward in a very short space of time?

The techniques I outline below have developed out of the constraints of time and the necessity to engage very quickly with a young person, knowing I may not see them again.

Initial contact

At our first meeting I find out if the young person knows why they are at the project and who referred them. I often read out the referral form to the young person and their parent/ carer to make sure that the information is correct. I initially see the young person with the parent/carer and encourage the adult to give me clear details about their concerns in front of the young person. Sometimes this is the only intervention needed.

Case study

A 13 year-old boy and his parents came to meet me about the death of his brother. His parents were very concerned about his lack of grief. The parents' telling of the story indicated that they had very different ways of coping with the death. One of them was processing their grief through a very open expression of their feelings, which the family found overwhelming. The other was managing their grief by thinking the issues through and distancing themselves from their feelings. The son was behaving like one of the parents and the concerns were primarily those of the other parent. They were able to acknowledge this and found some counselling for themselves as a couple about how to live with each other's very different ways of grieving.

When I see a young person I often draw a body outline and ask them to fill in their feelings using different colours (Marge Heegaard 1998). I use this to establish a baseline for me in terms of what their key feelings are, to affirm that a range of feelings in response to a death is usual, and to establish that words are not the only medium with which to communicate feelings. The young people I have worked with have been surprisingly open to drawing.

Case study

A 15 year old had experienced the recent death of a grandparent and was also managing the reawakening of his distress about the death of a parent. He filled in two body outlines for me, one on his feelings about his grandparent and the other with his feelings about the parental death. I referred to them in most of the sessions checking whether they had changed, and if they had, what had helped to change them. They were a clear visual way of showing this young person that he had changed and progressed significantly.

Affirming the grief reaction of the young person

Many young people are referred on the basis that they do not cry about the death. It is crucial that the young person and their parent/carer know that this is not unusual. Young people maybe too unsettled and fearful to cry, especially in front of another person. C.S. Lewis (1966) writes, 'No one ever told me that grief felt so like fear'. Young people are already managing turmoil as they experience adolescence; to compound this with the anxiety that grief may produce can be quite overwhelming. To cry you need to feel reasonably safe and secure.

Christ's (2000) research is very interesting in looking at the differences between early (12-14) and middle (15-17) adolescence. Early adolescents can have moments of acute grief and long periods of not expressing their grief. Again this needs to be affirmed and normalized.

Many young people feel they are getting it wrong and are worried that they are uncaring, unloving or pathetic. I try to normalize this by explaining it is very usual to be intensely critical of oneself following the death of someone close to you. I sometimes explain it as the 'catch 22' or double bind of grief.

Case study

I worked with a young woman who told me that she was pathetic and useless because she was overwhelmed and cried at school whenever she was reminded that her mother was dead. I helped her to reframe this by thinking of herself as someone who was sad because she loved and missed her mother.

I read Michael Rosen's *Sad Book* (Rosen and Blake 2004) with young people to illustrate the different ways grief can be managed. The *Sad Book* evocatively describes Michael Rosen's reactions to the death of his son and is beautifully illustrated by Quentin Blake. It reassures in its range of responses to bereavement and in the way Rosen so straightforwardly and openly describes how he manages his grief.

At Candle we give young people the Candle booklets 'Someone close to you has died' (2002) and 'Someone has died suddenly' (1999) to affirm the types of reactions they may have. Younger adolescents also like the little concertina leaflets 'A Pocket Book For Teenagers' and the 'Is This Normal?' poster from Bereavement Care in Staffordshire (Jordan and Rodway 1997).

Affirming the difference

Young people frequently talk about how different they feel to their peers since the death. Often they do not know other young people who are bereaved. Their whole world perspective changes when someone close to them has died. They can be irritated with the usual concerns of adolescence, finding it very offensive when other teenagers openly wish their parents were dead. They may feel the politics of the playground are trivial. They often need help with how to talk to their peers about the death and to be encouraged to verbalize their distress rather than act it out.

Dyregrov and Dyregrov (2008) refer to young people experiencing 'abrupt maturity' which leaves them with increased self-awareness but separates them from their peers. Their studies indicate that bereaved young people can experience personal growth and positive change.

Young people need to know that they are now seeing the world from a unique and different standpoint. This is out of the ordinary and is particularly hard on them because of their youth. However there are now valuable qualities about themselves that they would not have found if they had not experienced this death. I use the metaphor of a house with rooms that have never been opened. These rooms may initially be dark but with some exploration and light, these young people may discover things that they never knew existed. They can also, should they wish to, shut the doors of these rooms and return to ordinary adolescence.

Case study

I worked with a young woman whose father had died, who insisted she was different since his death and wanted to return to her old self. We explored the differences by looking at her attitudes and thoughts about other young people. She realised that her new compassion and understanding for other troubled young people was a consequence of the death of her father and was something to be valued. Once she had accepted this, she also began to find her old self again.

Open and transparent counselling

One of the aims of my work is to enable the young person to learn how to self-manage their grief. Their reaction to the death of someone close to them is of value and needs to be responded to with concern and interest. They can learn to manage and, if necessary, change this reaction.

The way that I convey this is by being open about the process that goes on inside me as I do the work. I talk about my different reactions to them, my choices about the work we are to do, and also my own struggle with emotion or not usually spoken about thoughts. Obviously I do this with an awareness of the context but I do it as genuinely as I can. The aim being to model:

- The usefulness of transparency about inner conflict when working out what to do
- The value of speaking out loud about feelings and thoughts even if it is anxiety provoking
- The range of feelings that are around when working on grief
- The lack of magic answers to the big issues in life like the death of someone close
- The importance of valuing inner uncertainty.

Case study

A young person whose father had died was very worried because he kept 'seeing' his father. I was open about my own uncertainty about what this was about and wondered out loud; was it a ghost or was the young person hallucinating? He acknowledged that he had thought about both explanations and both frightened him. I reassured him that bereaved people often think that they hear or 'see' the person who died. We explored his fears and the possible causes of either option. The hallucinations/ghost stopped after this session.

Being open about my feelings in response to being told about the death and not suppressing tears, fear, or anger models the safe expression of feelings. This needs to done in a way which also conveys a capacity to continue to be professional. Some young people need reassurance that they are not a burden or that their feelings are not destructive. They may previously have not expressed their grief to adults because of their fear of overwhelming them. It is vital to show the young person that it is possible to be okay and to have very powerful feelings.

Concern about wellbeing of parent/carer

It is reasonable and very common for young people to be concerned about their parent/carer's wellbeing. The ability of their adult carer to manage their caring role as well as their own grief has a large impact on the young person's well being (Christ 2000). However young people's expression of this concern may not be straightforward. They may act out their anxieties by being angry with the adult for expressing sadness, for example. Young people may come to counselling because of this concern about their adult carer and may need to talk about their fears and help to address them with the adult.

Young people may be very worried about their carer's mental or physical health or their financial situation. I ask for permission to share this worry with the adult concerned and advise on where they can get support if the anxiety is a valid one, or encourage the adult to offer reassurance if it is not.

Case study

A young man indicated how worried he was about his parent running up a huge credit card bill. He thought they would soon not be able to afford basic necessities. The parent had not appreciated how concerned her son was and took steps to manage this debt.

As with adults and younger children, many bereaved young people will be very sensitive to the possibility that those they are close to can die. They may not express their anxiety about this because part of their developmental task as adolescents is to separate from their parent or carer. They may want to avoid acknowledging dependency or to show that they care about their parent or carer. Parents and carers may need to be encouraged to broach this subject and to make open and clear arrangements for the care of the young person in the event of their death.

Clarifying and gathering information

When grieving we need to face the reality of what has happened and then manage our feelings about that reality (Worden 1991). Often young people do not know what has happened, or are muddled about significant events. This may be because no one has told them or because they did not want to hear at the time. Sometimes the death may have happened when they were younger and no one has since given them further, more age appropriate information.

The process of information gathering may be the most important part of the intervention with the young person. If in the sessions with the young person I am unclear about the events around the death, this will give me a clue about the things that need sorting out for the young person. I have used family trees and life event chronologies to help clarify what is really significant to the young person.

Case study

I worked with a young woman whose mother had died only a year previously. The young person talked about her as if she had died at least three years earlier. To try to resolve this,

I worked with the young woman on her life story and her family tree. I wrote out her life history as she described it to me and drew a geneogram of her family. We worked out that the significant issue for this young person was not actually the death but the very serious stroke her mother had had about three years earlier, and the subsequent life changes and loss of the parent she had known. The young person had not received any therapeutic help at this time and was still living with mixed feelings about her incapacitated mother and the relief she felt when she died. Those around her had assumed the issue was the death of her mother, whereas the young person's most burdensome feelings were guilt about the arguments they had had, and her lack of warm feelings towards her mother following the stroke.

If the death has been traumatic, the young person may not have been given all the information out of an adult concern to protect the young from the horrors of the world. This may leave young people with a sense of being excluded and not valued by the adults who care for them. The Childhood Bereavement Network video (2002) shows young people expressing very clearly and movingly how important it is to them to be included, when important information is being shared.

Case study

I have worked with a young person whose father committed suicide eight years previously and whose feelings had been reawakened by the subsequent death of another more distant relative. She knew that there was a note written by her father and that her mother had a copy, and she wanted to see the note. I encouraged her to ask her mother to see it. We then had a meeting with her mother at which she shared more information about the mode of death, which the young person had not known about. The family then contacted the coroner's officer and found out further details. This helped allay a longstanding fear of the young person that her father had committed suicide because of something she had done. The information from the inquest, the witness statements, and the suicide note all made it clear that this man committed suicide for other reasons, and that he had loved his children even though he had not seen them for a number of years prior to the death.

Sometimes the young person may not have information about the death because the adults do not have it either and part of the work is to enable the adults to find out any information that is available. It is easy to be so overwhelmed by the enormity of a death that we feel helpless and unable to be proactive. It can be helpful for the parent/carer concerned to do some information finding as this gives them a sense of being in control and in alliance with both the young person and the counsellor. They may need support to do this and some pointers about how to do it.

Case study

A 15 year-old girl had been told by a stranger that her father had died. Her mother had been separated from her father for most of this young person's life and had no contact with the father's family. She needed to find out the details of the death, so that the young person could deal with these instead of continuing to be in a state of uncertainty. The daughter had felt unable to ask her mother for fear of upsetting her. The mother needed to overcome her own feelings about this man she had left many years earlier. I did a piece of work with her about acknowledging her distress and her daughter's need for information. The mother made contact with the paternal extended family and her daughter appreciated having a link to family she had never known before, as well as finding out details about her father.

The use of bereavement models, writings, and research

Young people who come for bereavement counselling need help to make sense of their experience following the death. Developmentally they have the cognitive maturity to grasp sophisticated concepts and generally respond well to being given information about research, models and theories.

One model to which many young people respond positively is Stroebe's dual process model (Stroebe & Schut 1999). It is useful because it is a good visual tool and because it is a reassuring description of the grieving process. Christ's research (Christ 2000) indicates that early adolescents move between infrequent strong grief reactions and then long periods of carrying on as if nothing has changed. The dual process model describes how usual this is and also how helpful it is to have times where we focus on grief and times where we focus on other issues and the future. I have used this model when working with teenagers of all ages. I have drawn it and explained it to a young woman who was managing the sudden death of her best friend. It helped her to feel it was acceptable to be excited about going to university.

To my surprise I have found that C.S. Lewis' book (1966) about his grief when his wife died was felt to be really helpful by an older teenager who liked Lewis' description of the many internal conflicts she herself was feeling about her grief.

Colin Murray Parkes' (1972) work is very helpful as a straightforward description of the wide range of feelings that anyone may have following the death of someone close to them. Young people may need some basic education about these feelings. It can also be helpful to remind young people that many adults have explored and written about the mysteries and workings of grief without ever reaching a definitive answer. However what we do know is that it can have a bigger impact than we ever expected and that it can be survived well.

Working with a lack of response

Young people will rarely give you or the work you are doing with them a warm positive response. As a professional it is vital to remember that a lack of enthusiasm about the work we are doing with them, is not an indication of the impact we are having. If the young person turns up for sessions it probably means they feel hopeful about the work being fruitful. Even if they do not come this does not mean that they do not think the work is useful, it may just be that they cannot do the work at that time. They may come back later and it is worth giving the young person your contact details early on for this reason. Dyregrov & Dyregrov (2008) found that young people were not adept at informing people of their need for help and refused offers initially. They need repeated and sensitive offers of help and information about how to make contact.

Endings

The importance of an acknowledged ending cannot be overestimated. From the first session the young person will know that our work together is short term and how many sessions there will be. I will remind them regularly how many sessions are left. At the last session with a young person I will go through my notes and any body drawings to remind them of the work we have done, the changes that have happened and to give them feedback about their strengths and appreciations that I have of them. I will ask them to tell me the best thing about our work together and the most difficult thing. I will also help them think about the future and what they will do when they reach a bad patch. I will offer them the group for young people that we run (see Chapter 7) and remind them that they can always re refer themselves. I will also inform them of any local counselling services they could access in the future.

If they do not attend a last session, I will phone or write with some positive feedback and a reminder that they can come back.

Working with the professional network

Most young people are in contact with other professionals, the most common being school staff. I will make contact with schools to find out how young people are managing, to follow up a referral or to request that the school provide extra support or to liaise about information that we can share. Many schools have pastoral care systems with varyingly named professionals (learning mentors, counsellors, special educational needs coordinators, school nurses, tutors, year heads, family liaison officers or chaplains) who will follow up my concerns about the long term support needs of a bereaved young person. I may also need to liaise with other counselling agencies, family doctors, Child and Adolescent Mental Health Services, Youth Offending Teams, Social Services and the Police. Many young people and their families are daunted by the complex systems in many organisations so need the Candle Project to find a named contact with whom they can relate.

Conclusion

We have offered our experience of working in a particular context and within a limited time frame with children, young people and families. We have outlined how our approaches influence the work and hope to have conveyed key issues of connecting quickly with children and young people in ways that make sense of their experience, using a variety of techniques.

We would emphasize that we prioritise building alliances with our clients whether they be individual young people or whole families. We do this by focusing on their concerns and also reminding them of their strengths and highlighting how well they have survived thus far.

Sometimes our families arrive with a belief that a death will disable them forever unless they can learn to 'get over it'. Our view is that young people and families will have gained skills and abilities they may never have learned otherwise and may not yet have recognized. Our hope is that irrespective of the techniques chosen the work can support the creativity of families and young people in adjusting to a new future.

References

Burnham, J. (1992) Approach, method, technique: making distinctions and creating connections. *Human Systems*, **3**(1): 3–26.

Childhood Bereavement Network VHS/DVD (2002) *A death in the Lives of ...* London: National Children's Bureau.

Christ, G. (2000) *Healing children's Grief: Surviving a Parent's Death From Cancer*. Oxford: Oxford University Press.

Crossley, D. (2000) *Muddles, Puddles and Sunshine Activity Book*. Winston's Wish/ Hawthorn Press.

Dyregrov, K. and Dyregrov, A. (2008) *Effective Grief and Bereavement Support: The Role of Family, Friends, Colleagues, Schools and Support Professionals*. London and Philadelphia: Jessica Kingsley.

Freeman, J. Epston, D. and Lobovits, D. (1997) *Playful Approaches to Serious Problems: Narrative Therapy with Children and Their Families*. New York: Norton.

Heegaard, M. (1988) *When Someone Very Special Dies: Children can Learn to Cope With Grief*. Minneapolis, MN: Woodland Press.

Jordan, G. and Rodway, K. (1999a) *A Pocket Book for Teenagers*. Staffordshire Bereavement Care.

Jordan, G. and Rodway, K. (1997b) *Is This Normal?* Staffordshire Bereavement Care.

Klass, D., Silverman, P.R., and Nickman, S. (eds) (1996) *Continuing Bonds: New Understandings of Grief*. Washington DC: Taylor & Francis.

Lewis, C.S. (1966) *A Grief Observed*. London: Faber and Faber Ltd.

Lewis, P. and Kavanagh, C. (1995) Play as dialogue, giving voice to the child in family therapy. *Human Systems*, **6** (3–4): 227–41.

Nadeau, J.W. (1998) *Families Making Sense of Death*. California: Sage.

Neimeyer, R. (2001) *Meaning Reconstruction and the Experience of Loss*. Washington DC: American Psychological Association.

Parkes, C.M. (1972) *Bereavement: Studies of Grief in Adult Life*. New York: International Universities Press.

Rowling, L. (2003) *Grief in School Communities: Effective Support Strategies*. Oxford: Oxford University Press.

St Christopher's Candle Project (1999) *Someone Has Died Suddenly*. London: St Christopher's Hospice.

St Christopher's Candle Project (2002) *Someone Close to You Has Died*. London: St Christopher's Hospice.

Stokes, J. (2004). *Then, Now and Always: Supporting Children as They Journey Through Grief: A Practitioner's Guide*. Cheltenham: Winston's Wish.

Stokes, J. (2007) Resilience and bereaved children; helping a child to develop a resilient mind-set following the death of a parent. In: Monroe, B. and Oliviere, D. (eds). *Resilience in Palliative Care: Achievement in Adversity*. Oxford. Oxford University Press pp. 39–66.

Stroebe, M. and Schut, H. (1999) The dual process model of coping with bereavement: rationale and description. *Death Studies 99*, **23** (3): 197–224.

Walsh, F. McGoldrick, M. (1995) *Living Beyond Loss: Death in the Family*. New York: Norton.

Walter, T. (1999) *On bereavement: the culture of grief*. Oxford: Oxford University Press.

White, M. (1989) Saying hullo again: the incorporation of the lost relationship in the resolution of grief. In: White, M. (ed) *Selected Papers*. Adelaide:Dulwich Centre Publications.

White, M. and Epston, D. (1990) Externalizing of the problem. In White, M. (ed). *Narrative Means to Therapeutic Ends*. New York: Norton, pp. 38–76.

White, M. Delight and the unexpected. Workshop 14.6.01-15.6.01 held at School of Oriental and African Studies, University of London, offered by the Brief Therapy Practice.

Wilson, J. (1998) *Child-focused Practice: A Collaborative Systemic Approach*. London: Karnac.

Worden, J.W. (1991) *Grief Counselling and Grief Therapy: A Handbook for the Mental Health Practitioner* (2nd ed.) New York: Springer.

Worden, J.W. (1996) *Children and Grief: When a Parent Dies*. New York: Guilford Press.

Chapter 7

Groupwork

Patsy Way, Frances Kraus, and the Candle Team

You gotta connect because it means a lot to
communicate with people.
*(Personal reflections from a teenager who was part
of a bereavement group run by the Candle Project at
St Christopher's Hospice)*

Bereavement can be a very isolating experience and children have told us that
they did not believe anyone else in their school had experienced a significant
bereavement, although McCarthy and Jessup (2005 p1) suggest that the vast
majority of children and young people will be bereaved of someone important
in their lives before they leave school.

Why groups?

Groups for the bereaved at any age can play a significant role in supporting
people feeling alone and isolated after a death (Dyregrov and Dyregrov 2008b).

There are many possible models of groupwork coming from a variety of
psychotherapeutic traditions notably the practice of Yalom (Yalom and Leszcz
2005) and psychodrama (Moreno 1989) in the US and Foulkes (1964) in the
UK. Some of the group aims identified by these theorists, such as the recognition of the importance of sharing a common experience, the offering of hope
and information, and the idea that group members often achieve a greater level
of self-awareness through interacting with others, are reflected in children's
bereavement groups being organized currently in the UK.

The literature describes examples of ongoing, closed groups meeting for a
fixed number of sessions, which have a psychodynamic theoretical base
(Lohnes and Kalter 1994; Smith and Pennells 1995; Kirk and McManus 2002;

Pfeffer et al. 2002). A model of residential weekend camps exemplified by Winston's Wish (Stokes 2004) has gained popularity, focusing as these camps do on a non-pathologizing notion of support for grieving families as distinct from a directly therapeutic model.

Groups at the Candle Project

The Candle Project has developed an ever evolving programme of group interventions, growing organically from requests made by the families we work with and our own experiments in addressing a perceived need. Our catchment area, which consists of a mixture of inner city and suburban districts with a high proportion of families from socially deprived backgrounds, necessitated a pragmatic approach to the structuring of our groupwork programme. We have always offered one-off groups, as previous experience has taught us that this is the level of commitment we can reasonably expect from the families we work with. Some of these groups are offered on an on-going basis, as will be described later, but none of our groups have a closed membership, so newcomers are always able to join at the first opportunity. Each new group is piloted to assess whether it fulfils the identified need. All groups continue in a process of constant re-evaluation through dialogue with users, staff and volunteers to ensure we are focusing our energies in an effective and appropriate way. Groups have particular needs and issues but the stated aims remain the same; facilitating growth and enabling new strategies for meeting the changes and challenges following bereavement.

Aims for Candle Project groups

The aims are:

- to give children/young people the chance to meet others in the same situation as themselves. Grief can be a very isolating experience.
- to help them learn some new ways to express their feelings about what has happened and give them a chance to do so.
- to provide an opportunity for children/young people to ask questions and share some of their memories about the person who died.
- to offer their parents and carers the opportunity to meet others in the same situation.

Volunteers

All individual and family interventions are delivered by the paid Candle team, but the groupwork programme has always relied on volunteers, who work with staff to offer 22 group events a year at the time of writing. Candle has a team of 25 volunteers, some of whom have been with the project since it began and we operate a rolling programme to train small groups of new applicants, most of who work as staff or volunteers for the hospice. Volunteers need ongoing training and support, (Chapter 14) which makes demands on staff time, and this needs to be incorporated into the planning, preparation and reflection time involved in delivering a group.

We rely on our trained volunteers to demonstrate a sensitive understanding of the very practical as well as the emotional needs of children or young people. This demands a flexibility which might, for example, involve a volunteer in playing football with a child and then ten minutes later be deep in discussion with the same boy about the effect on him of his father's suicide.

It is crucial to ensure that volunteers are very clear about the specific goals in devising the programme and are comfortable in what is being asked of them. In training and planning meetings, we rehearse a proposed activity which allows them an opportunity to feed back their experience of it, and any reservations they may have can be addressed. Volunteers are then able to use their own experience in leading and supporting the children/young people. They bring different perspectives and will sometimes raise helpful questions and challenge Candle staff quite vigorously about the purpose and value of an exercise, often being concerned whether an activity will distress the participants too much. They sometimes worry about talking directly to children and young people about death, dying and existential questions and careful explanation is needed to show why we think it important and how this relates to the aims of the groups.

Most groups involve volunteers in working with a particular age group but in the Younger Children's Group and the Family Workshop we engage parents/carers and children together, and volunteers need support in managing this different dynamic. They sometimes need to be coached, using role plays and discussion, to work alongside adults caring for bereaved young children. It is necessary for volunteers to understand the importance of modelling ways of talking with the children so that adult carers can feel supported and enabled to elaborate and develop conversations with their children about the bereavement.

Development of the group programme

The project, which celebrated its tenth anniversary in 2008, emerged in response to expressed interest from local community groups who wanted a supportive service for all bereaved children in the area, whether connected to the hospice or not. In addition to brief individual intervention and family support offered by Candle staff, it was thought important that children have a chance to meet others in similar circumstances.

The children's group days began in 1998. As the team grew in size, we were able to respond to the different needs of children of different ages, and began the young people's groups in 1999 and groups for younger children in 2005.

Support to parents and carers is also part of our stated aims. The Parent/Carers Group emerged in 1999 at the specific request of families who had received support from the Candle Project and wished to continue to support one another on a regular basis (see Chapter 20). After this group had become well established there was seen to be a need for those more recently bereaved to meet, facilitated by a team member, to work with some of the very raw feelings following recent bereavement. The Monthly Bereavement Group began in 2003. Then about two years ago, it was noted that the project was receiving referrals from a very invisible group in the community, namely older siblings who were caring for younger brothers and sisters, sometimes after sudden and traumatic bereavements and having to struggle with critical financial, housing and legal worries as well as continuing to work and study and establish their own lives. The Sibling Carer Group was initiated in 2006 to support these young people.

More recently in 2008, the Candle team offered a Family Workshop day in response to requests from the Parent/Carer Group for more specific input on parenting issues and the team's reflections on the work of Sandler and Ayers (2002).

Children and families bereaved by suicide or murder presented us with particular issues. We wished to offer them their own group, particularly as, of all families suffering bereavement, these types of death are often surrounded by the greatest silence. Ideally we would have liked to offer them a separate group experience. For example, Winston's Wish organize specific weekends for families bereaved by murder or suicide (Stokes 2004). However our project would not have sufficient numbers to support this so that some families would have to wait many months until we had enough people to offer a group for a given age range. The team spent a great deal of time deliberating how to enable these families to meet and have a voice, talking with others about their experiences. We had some concerns about the effects on others of hearing these children recounting their family stories of murder and suicide. Eventually we decided to experiment by including this group of families in the Children's Group. The issues raised were enormously thought provoking for the adults involved, but children took it in their stride and we have continued this inclusive practice in all the groups.

Practicalities

Most groups are held on Saturdays when children, families and volunteers are more available and the hospice space is also freer. The Young People's group meets three times a year on Tuesday evenings between 6.30pm and 9pm because they preferred not to meet on Saturdays, when they are busy with part time jobs, clubs and other activities.

Some groups, such as the days for children, can only be offered for a single session as this is what can be managed within the team's resources. Other groups such as the Parent/Carers, Sibling Carers and Young People's Groups are able to meet in an ongoing way, three times a year. In this way some families are able to maintain continued connections with the project and the team can engage at different levels at different times with children, young people or families who may need and value ongoing support over time. Thus, a recently bereaved mother might be offered the adult bereavement group while her three children are invited to the Teenage Evening Group (13+ years), the Children's Day (8–12 years) and the Younger Children's Day (3–7 years)[1] respectively. Subsequently, the whole family might come together to a Family Workshop.

Typically referrals come from Candle staff members who have been working with a child/children and family. On occasion other external professionals will have worked with a child or young person and refer them on to us for a group experience.

Throughout, the project has had to work within very tight and pragmatic frameworks. Offering group days depends heavily on the generosity of St Christopher's Hospice in affording space in larger rooms and the garden to accommodate us. We are also able to offer transport to and from groups for those needing it and appropriate refreshment depending on the time of day.

Managing the day

The groups require careful preparation and team management of tasks. Dates are planned months in advance and the rooms are booked. Administration time is taken in the writing and sending of invitations, the monitoring of responses, and the drawing up of lists of participants expected. After a group, numbers attending and feedback information are also logged by the administrator.

With the exception of the Bereavement Group and the Parent/Carer's Group, a planning meeting is held with staff and volunteers in the week before the group. This meeting has two objectives, namely to manage the practical preparations

---

[1] A judgement would need to be made about the appropriateness of the group for very young children. In general, children able to talk and express themselves in play would be ready for the type of group experience we have devised.

and focus the working group on the purpose of the day or evening. Preparation tasks include finalizing the programme, delegating tasks and preparing any equipment necessary. Time is allowed before a group event to set it up and afterwards to tidy away.

After the group the staff and volunteer group reconvene for a supervisory session in which they can reflect on issues emerging, voice any concerns about particular children or young people, and evaluate the whole experience. Procedures are also in place to address any possible concerns about keeping a child safe. In the month following a group, the staff involved also have a supervision session.

The Children's Group (8-12 years)

Joel listened quietly to Sam's description of the days leading up to his mother's death. Barely perceptibly, he nudged the box of tissues on the table towards Sam when he saw tears rising. Joel had been the first child to take a turn in the group to tell the story of his bereavement; his father's suicide. This was the first time either boy had told the story of the death in their family to a peer. By the end of the day, after a mixture of serious, playful, focused and energetic activities, the boys were friends and asked their parents if they might keep in touch with each other.

For children like Joel and Sam, such a day holds an opportunity to develop a sense of themselves, and their place in their family and the wider world following the death of someone important to them. They will have a chance to reflect on events and the changes that followed the death. They can remember the person who died through ritual and creative means and explore their own feelings in relation to some momentous changes in their lives. Above all they will have met others who have also experienced bereavement.

Grace Christ (2000) has focused attention on the impact of bereavement at particular ages and stages of development. Her findings address a different cultural context and bereavement of a parent from cancer. However it provides a fascinating snapshot of issues raised by children in this age group. Christ notes that, though many feel guilt about the death, they can think through and respond to explanations, having developed more concrete operational (logical) thinking by this age. Although children may actively express a wish for the dead person to return, they have had more experience of the world than younger siblings and are better able to cognitively appreciate the finality of death. They are also more likely to have the language and experience to ask for information and sometimes actively seek out and engage adults who might offer it. They were more likely to engage in anticipatory grief when the death was expected than younger children.

As with many children, the experience of the death opened up anxieties about the possibility of other losses and brought forth fears for themselves and other family members. She notes that their emotional reactions tended to be more muted than in other age groups. The Children's Group attempts to address this area in a variety of ways with a range of activities. The day aims to be a coherent experience to widen and deepen a child's understanding and offer the possibility of sharing his/her experience with others.

Volunteers and staff work from 9am to 5pm, though the children meet between 10.30am and 3.30pm. The day begins with explanations, welcoming activities and the decorating of a memory box which the child carries through the day, adding objects made in different activities. There is then a warm-up game and introductions. Children split into smaller groups and play a card game which allows the group to get to know one another better, focusing on their likes and dislikes and interests. Having become familiar with the group, children are invited to show a photo of the person(s) who died and tell their story. This would be modelled initially by the adults facilitating the group. This can be a deeply connecting and moving experience (as described above) for children who may never have had this opportunity with peers.

Through the day, the small group will have a chance to engage together in a range of activities. There will be an opportunity for remembering, perhaps in the making of a memory jar (Stokes 2004 p114) or memory stones (an exercise adapted from the rough rocks activity (Crossley and Stokes 2002). Feelings can be explored through activities using colour association such as collage or the colouring of feelings in a drawing of one's body (Heegaard 1988) to locate and identify specific emotions. Children discuss who and what might help with difficult feelings.

Children are invited to ask a doctor questions to facilitate understanding of the causes of the death but the discussion sometimes broadens to include current concerns children have about their own health and safety and that of their carers. For example, in a recent group the doctor was pressed with many questions about addictive behaviours (smoking, alcohol, drugs) from children concerned about their remaining carers.

The day also includes a short candle-lighting ritual in which children are often very focused and emotionally expressive. There is also lunch and activities encouraging fun and energy-release such as parachute games and a treasure hunt. We include an art or music activity to encourage other means of expression. This connects with thinking behind the Dual Process Model developed by Stroebe and Schut (1999) who argued the usefulness in oscilating in bereavement between loss oriented activities, such as our candlelighting ritual, and the sadness evoked in telling the story of the death, and more restoration oriented opportunities inviting release from tensions, and more forward-thinking, future-oriented activities addressing the challenges faced in a changed world.

While the children are involved in group activities, parent-carers have an opportunity to meet in a group facilitated by Candle staff and volunteers to discuss their common issues and changes in their lives.

The Young People's Group (13-18 years)

Case study

Helen is describing her own and her parents' grief reaction to the sudden death of her older brother. She insists it is impossible to tell her parents how she feels; they're already too upset and overwhelmed by their own grief. Sonia has a similar story and they acknowledge they feel they have lost their parents to grief. The group leader asks if anybody has shared their grief with their parent or carer. David describes sitting with his mum, after his dad died, and the two of them crying over old family photographs. His mum was fine afterwards, and he feels closer to her now. Helen and Sonia listen carefully. In the large group they make collages of images which remind them of their brothers. Back in the small group they talk about their collages and how they will show their parents. They have been reassured that they are not alone and that it is possible to get support from grieving parents.

With an average attendance of 25, this is an open group of young people with a wide range of experience of bereavement, some deaths taking place only months previously and others over ten years before. Some deaths were unexpected and traumatic, others anticipated and timely. Some young people come from very affluent backgrounds, others are very economically deprived. More than a third are male and the group represents a wide range of ethnic origins, cultures and religions.

From ongoing experience of the group and following suggestions from a young people's user group facilitated by Candle in 2005, we have developed an organizational model for structuring the group. We learnt that different young people appreciate different aspects of the group. Some prefer small groups or informal times for games and refreshment while others prefer the large group and more structured activities. Some like to listen to others' experiences, others like to tell their stories and be heard.

We begin with semi-structured activities; games and quizzes, a welcome in the large group, and a name game as warming up activities. Then, so the young people can tell their bereavement story, for about 20 minutes we have them in small groups of four or five with two adults. The young people who have attended before are encouraged to start, to model being open and courageous enough to talk about the death and its impact.

There follows a large group activity which varies each time. This may involve creative activities such as pictures or poems associated with memories or feelings about the person who died. Some activities practice coping strategies, for example role playing the management of sadness or other strong feelings. The young people have taken photographs to illustrate mutual group support and the hospice digital arts therapist has photographed them as they remembered the person who has died. Other sessions focused on music, relaxation, and other creative ways to express and release anger and frustration. Nurses, doctors and police officers have talked to them about their roles and answered questions about a death.

After the large group activity, the young people go back to their original small group to explore and integrate their experience. Finally for the last 30 minutes we provide food and they socialize and complete feedback forms.

The feedback is usually very positive about at least one aspect of the group. For example: *I found the small group helpful. It lets you know you are not alone* or *I liked the remembering card. It made me do thinking I haven't done in a long time.*

Many young people return many times to the group. Some of them greatly value an ongoing link with the project over several years and this allows the team to monitor their needs and progress. The ratio of adults to young people is usually about one to two. This means we can be very responsive and catch up individually with those who may have been through a particularly difficult time, possibly involving further loss and change, or if we notice a young person looking distressed. For example, a young person originally attending the group because a sibling had died needed extra support following the death of a friend. We can also follow up any significant concerns we may have if a young person is feeling suicidal or is at risk of harm.

The group also thrives because the young people attending are courageous enough to come, are open to trying out the activities, and are compassionate towards one another. It is a privilege to be part of this and to be reminded of the resilience and capacity of young people to face and support one another.

The Younger Children's Group (3-7 years)

Case study

Jermain was three years old and his mother had died following a road traffic crash. He and his sister had been told about the ambulance that came to collect his mother and take her to the hospital and the doctors and nurses who had tried to make her better. 'And then she went to heaven' affirmed Jermain as this is how adults caring for him had explained it, in a manner that invited no further questions or discussion.

Dyregrov has discussed young children's understanding of bereavement (2008a p12–32). Christ (2000) has outlined her research findings on the effects of bereavement in the young children in her study and described (p46) play, drawings, and symbolic play as the 'lingua franca' of this age group. She defines the key issues for very young children as being around understanding the permanence of death and their difficulties in facing strong emotions from parents, perhaps of intense rage or sadness. She points out that at the upper end of this age group, at seven, children's worlds have often widened greatly and they have a much broader understanding.

Jermain and his father Leroy came to a group for younger children. They were welcomed by Rita, a trained and experienced volunteer, who sat down with them to explain the plan for the day. She answered Leroy's questions while engaging Jermain in decorating his memory box (Stokes 2004 p80). She explained that he would be invited to visit different play areas with his father and in each area he would gain a stamp on his card. She took them into the 'Home and School' area which was set out with small tables and play materials. Jermain and his father were invited to co-create memories (see Chapter 10) of his mother doing ordinary household tasks like making phone calls and collecting him from pre-school. His father gradually became more involved and, encouraged by Rita and another volunteer, they moved on to a 'Medical' play area where nurses in uniform and a doctor explained what paramedics and hospital staff would have done to try to save his mother. Sadly, they could not stop her dying, though hospitals often can save people. Next they visited the 'Living and Dying' area where Jermain stared at the two goldfish in the bowl and talked to John, another volunteer, about how he could tell that the goldfish were alive because they were swimming and eating. He and Leroy then joined in the 'burial' of a dead spider and fly in a tray adapted as a cemetery and planted flowers at the little graves. John also explained that some people, like Jermain's mother, are cremated rather than buried. They are very carefully burnt and all the ashes collected in a jar or box. Jermain filled a little jar with sand, which has a texture similar to ashes and labelled it 'my mum' and added it to his memory box. John explained that when someone dies their body cannot feel anything so nothing hurts anymore. They cannot see, hear, feel, or eat.

Jermain looked puzzled. 'How did my mum get to heaven then?' Leroy looked to John for help. John showed him a collection of sacred books and artifacts and explained that many people have thought about that for a long time and had lots of different ideas but nobody was able to tell us directly after they died. Some people think people go to heaven, some think they just stop existing, and some people say they don't know. John explained that it seems that heaven is not a place like London that you can visit in a car or even a rocket. It is a very difficult question but it connects to how we remember that person and how they become part of our thoughts in the future.

The day progressed with activities for the children focusing on remembering the person, which included a short candle-lighting ritual as well as fun and energetic activities. Leroy welcomed the chance to join other parents and carers for coffee and sandwiches followed by a discussion led by a Candle staff member and volunteer. The group had been very moved by their experiences of talking in this way through play with their children, and it had raised questions and memories for them.

Setting up and clearing away the play areas for this group involves a lot of equipment. Volunteers need support and training to develop skills in welcoming families, explaining the programme and inviting them into a creative mood of playful engagement. Parents/ carers may need varying levels of support and encouragement to relax and participate.

This is our response in a particular area of London to the needs of younger children at this time. In the period we have been running the groups, we have made many modifications, and worked with and learnt from our volunteers. The rationale for the day derives from a belief that younger children can engage with the complexities of life and death (Dyregrov 2008a, Way Chapter 10) and play is the most appropriate learning vehicle for this age group (Sunderland 2007). Our purpose in structuring the group in this way is to help children understand and make sense of the events surrounding a death and the consequent changes, and support families in developing a story of what has happened which may support their moving on. Hopefully these are practical beginnings for conversations which can continue at home.

The Parent/Carer Self Help Group

Candle staff and volunteers provide the practical support that makes this group happen. The group itself is described in Chapter 20, and further information about how to set up a parent/carer self help group based on the experiences at Candle can be obtained or downloaded from the Childhood Bereavement Network website,[www.childbereavementnetwork.org.uk].

There had been clear messages from parents and carers from the outset of the project about the need for a forum which would offer ongoing contact and support. In 1999, two parents who were also part of the Candle Advisory Group decided to start a group for others in a similar situation to themselves, i.e single parents through bereavement. Candle was able to undertake the administration, which involves sending out invitations, booking rooms and transport if necessary, and most importantly providing volunteer childcare. Parent/carer childcare was added to the list of tasks and groups we expected volunteers to help with. The emphasis is childcare; we are entertaining and occupying the children for the two hour period the group runs, and this provides an opportunity for volunteers to use skills and talents that may not be used in the other groups. Volunteers offer craft activities, games, and a trip to the park for some form of physical activity, weather permitting. The group of trained volunteers are often joined by individuals, usually staff or volunteers from St Christopher's, who are interested in becoming a Candle volunteer, as the childcare gives them a brief taster of the Candle groups in a supervised environment with a staff member always present.

The volunteers are co-ordinated by a Candle team member, who also provides supervision for the two parents who run the group. Many of the children have been attending for some time and know one another quite well. They show a remarkable level of tolerance and acceptance of one another's differences, and appreciate the amount of adult attention available during the group. The adult:child ratio is usually 1:2, and sometimes as high as 1:1, which is unusual for many children in families where a parent has died.

The group provides an opportunity for volunteers to engage with fun activities with bereaved children, and get to know them without the anxieties of the other group events, which have very tight timetables for activities.

Case study

This group allows children to connect to peers, volunteers and Candle staff in a very informal way. For example, Patrick and his two older brothers enjoyed meeting others in this way once a term. Patrick enjoyed playing games with volunteers he had met originally at a Younger Children's Group and who worked with him again later in the Family Workshop. He was also able to touch base with the Candle staff member who had worked with the family initially and he found it easy to request a session with her later, under the extended warranty (Kraus Chapter 11) as he had been playing and chatting with her while his mother attended the Parent/Carer group.

The monthly bereavement group for parents

To walk into a room full of strangers on your own in unfamiliar surroundings may take some courage at the best of times. To walk into the same situation as a recently bereaved carer can feel totally overwhelming. Sandra panicked when she drove up to the hospice to attend a bereavement group, returning home immediately, before even getting out of her car. Only after replaying a voicemail message inviting her to the group did she decide to return, driven by a desperate need to break the isolation of bereavement and meet with other parents who could understand her pain.

As part of a bereavement project working with children and families, we had become only too aware of the isolation often involved in lone parenting while grieving. Our Children's Group day allows us to run a facilitated session for parents (and any other primary carers) during the morning, and these one off sessions frequently highlighted the need for ongoing support, particularly for those newly bereaved.

By September 2003, five years into the project, we were able to set up a group for parents, to give them time to talk together in a supportive environment. It complemented the Parent/Carer Self-Help Group, providing a more frequent and regular experience of meeting. It meets from ten o'clock to midday monthly on a weekday morning. This allows time for parents to deliver children to school as we do not have resources to offer childcare.

Parents initially receive some information about the group from the referring member of the team. The Candle staff member coordinating the group phones them to discuss any fears they may have and to reassure them about the support and safety of the group.

The group is run by a staff member and a volunteer. Another volunteer also meets and greets parents as we know this is important in engaging newcomers.

Although the group is aimed at the more recently bereaved, we have been flexible where parents have had little contact, if any, with other bereaved parents and are actively seeking this connection. We also acknowledge that grief has no particular timetable and allow members to stay within reasonable time limits, usually for up to a year. Only once, when numbers of referrals increased significantly did we suggest carers move on to our Parent/Carer Group. Otherwise members have left at a point when they feel able to leave, attending the self help group if they wish to.

When new members join the group they introduce themselves, talk about their children, and name the person who has died. Confidentiality rules are stated and people are invited to disclose information about themselves at a level that is comfortable for them. The group have taken responsibility for exchanging contact details and the practice of sharing texts and e-mails has proved very supportive between group meetings. For example, some members have experienced difficulty sleeping and e-mailing one another at night has been very reassuring. This process of communication has allowed members to share their difficulties and retain their humour. One current member has the ability to text jokes.

Group members have supported and advised one another on issues such as schooling and childcare. Some members who have been through the anniversary of the death and other significant events have enabled those more recently bereaved to imagine how it may be for them. This has been invaluable in supporting their parenting skills, and has helped some in the group to feel that they are doing more than just coping. They have shared practical advice about cooking easy nourishing meals, establishing sleep routines, and managing discipline as well as offering ideas for making time to enjoy being together as a new kind of family.

One parent talked about feeling guilty that his son had not gone to the Catholic secondary school his wife would have preferred. Talking through the options, which had changed since her death, allowed him to see that he had made the best decision given his current circumstances and the group has been supportive in affirming decisions that might previously have been taken jointly with a partner.

Bereaved carers have often commented that others feel threatened by the intensity of their grief and therefore often avoid them. Under the stresses of bereavement, family relationships and friendships can be very strained, some-times to the point of collapse. The group can offer empathy and understanding in a non-judgmental environment in which members are listened to respectfully. Despite wide-ranging differences between members in cultural, religious and socio-economic terms, this may be the only space for these parents to share their feelings and talk to others in a similar situation.

As Dave, a member of the group commented, *It reassures me that I am not living in a world of my own. I am not unique in this.*

The sibling carer's group

The Candle Siblings Group is an open group for siblings who are caring for younger brothers and sisters following the death of a parent. Sometimes the parent who died was a single parent, sometimes there is another parent but s/he is unwilling or unable to care for the family.

These sibling carers (see Chapter 19), who are often young themselves (aged 17 – late 20's), have particular needs that distinguish them from other family groups. The Candle Project found in 2006 that staff were seeing a few young sibling carers who did not fit into the Parent/Carers bereavement groups but were experiencing a desire to meet. In the same way as all our groups have devel-oped, we responded to a need and set up an initial pilot meeting alongside the Parent/Carer Group. This proved successful and has continued since then.

Case study

For example, a 21 year old woman Ananya and her brother Amar aged 9 experienced the deaths of both mother and father within a 12 month period. Their extended family were abroad, and Ananya was faced with sorting out the family home and finances and supporting her brother, who had learning difficulties and struggled at school. Both were grieving deeply and their relationship became quite fragile and difficult. The Candle worker discussed alternative care arrangements with them and considered a referral to social care services, but with her help and support their determination to stay together as a family was rewarded, and Amar has now made a successful secondary school transfer.

For many siblings becoming a carer means putting on hold their own education, careers and relationships, and sometimes results in a need to move house and change the children's school arrangements. They find themselves taking on a parental role and so having to negotiate new relationships, boundaries, discipline, and routines. Suddenly taking on the role of parent to your brothers and sisters puts tremendous pressure on grieving young people, who may be quite vulnerable. Learning how to parent emerges as a huge challenge, and at times causes a lot of conflict and confusion of roles.

These young people also trying to deal not only with their own grief, but that of their siblings also, and at times this can be overwhelming. In addition these sibling carers are often facing legal, financial and social/housing issues, some of which are extremely difficult and stressful. They need to liaise with social care services, schools, solicitors and often the legal system, and receive little if any support with this. In many cases they are also acting as the link to extended family, both in this country and abroad, and this can involve certain expectations from other family members as to how they should parent their siblings.

By setting up a group for these carers, we were attempting to address some of the particular issues that made them distinct from other carers, acknowledge and value what they are doing, and also to support them at a vulnerable time. The purpose of setting up the group was to give these carers an opportunity to meet and support one another, to share common experiences and to offer advice and guidance where possible. The emotional support appeared to be as important as any practical advice we could give.

Membership is very transient and people come and go depending on their circumstances, which is to be expected with such a young group. The members take ownership of the group and need to access it when it is beneficial to them, whether that is only once or over a longer period. The shape and feel of the group is informal, yet very concrete guidance can be accessed. We aim to facilitate an open and welcoming environment, making it possible for these sibling carers, who feel isolated and weighed down with responsibility, to come and share their experiences.

The group meets three times a year at St Christopher's Hospice at the same time as the Parent-Carer Group so that childcare is available for these younger siblings. A staff facilitator was proposed initially with the idea that the group might evolve into a self-help group. This facilitator has to date stayed with the group, as this takes some pressure off these already busy young people by helping shape and structure the sessions for them. Group members have told us that they prefer this arrangement. The group usually starts with introductions and an opportunity to briefly share their story and then there is time to look at specific issues such as managing childcare and discipline, having time for themselves, and having space for their own friends and close relationships.

We have been able to bring in other professionals to give advice and guidance. For example, through a partnership with the Family Rights Group, a national charity that advises families whose children are involved with or require social care services, a member of the welfare team in the hospice has been invited to advise on benefits and members of the group are contributing to an initiative to improve the support available to sibling carers nationally.

The strength of the group is in the validation it provides for members, always emphasizing the positive while validating their very difficult and particular experiences. Many of the carers describe feeling very low emotionally, and receive little positive feedback, appreciation, or acknowledgment for their efforts. Group members are able to give one another positive feedback and encouragement.

Participants say that they find the experience invaluable and supportive, and they are keen to express that, however hard their new role is, it is worth it. One carer wrote at the outset of the sibling group;

Case study

'In a new situation, when meeting people, I often find it difficult explaining my circumstances. I've just started at Uni and it's such a heavy thing to say "I look after my sister" when I've just met them. I've been to Candle and done groups with parents but didn't think there were other siblings out there doing this job like me. I think it would be really beneficial to meet others like me and share stories, difficulties and ideas'.

There is a sense of relief that other young people are experiencing something similar and the complexity of all the issues is not so odd or overwhelming but normal and expected. They are all adjusting to becoming a new kind of family.

The Family Workshop

The idea for a family workshop to complement the other groups run by the Candle Project arose both from an expressed wish from members of the existing Parent/ Carers Group for more structured activities or workshops to help with the practicalities of parenting and also from our own perceptions, as practitioners, of the needs of the group.

Although within the project we work primarily with children or young people there is always a dialogue with parents or carers and sometimes the work focuses on opening up the channels of communication between children and their parents or carers. At other times there is a need for specific interventions with parents especially where, pre-bereavement, there were already existing stresses in managing the dynamics of family life. Parents and carers can be stretched beyond their capacity to cope in the weeks and months following the death of a family member. Newly reconstituted families struggle to manage day-to-day life as well as new roles and the place for free time is often overlooked. Yet both children and parents or carers need time away from relentless grieving (Stroebe and Schut 1999), so practical strategies and guidance are often needed by both parents and children. Our initial thinking around the family workshop was also underpinned by the shift in UK service provision towards a whole-family approach to mental health work enshrined in the 2004 Every Child Matters – Agenda for Change for Children programme. Here, the part that parents, carers and families play in ensuring positive outcomes for children is clearly defined; promotion of healthy choices and positive behaviour, provision of safe and stable homes and support in learning and being economically active.

An evidential rationale was provided by the research and work carried out by the Family Bereavement Programme (FBP) run by Irwin Sandler and Tim Ayers (2002) at the Preventative Research Centre at Arizona State University. At the Candle Project, we decided to focus our Family Workshop Day in 2008 on developing listening and communication skills and exploring how to find a place in the week for fun family time. Activities for children and young people were planned to run parallel to a workshop for their parents and carers with a joint workshop where everyone came together at the end of the day.

The children's activities were organized according to age which broadly corresponded to the ages of our existing children's groups, that is, four to seven, eight to twelve and thirteen to eighteen. A range of different activities around the themes of listening and communicating effectively was planned. Parents and carers spent the morning as a group with one of the volunteers experienced in running groups and a parent who has used the service and who has herself experienced in running training days. This flattening of the distinction between professionals and service users connects to the Candle team's commitment to service user involvement.

Here the emphasis was on improving listening skills, and we invited the parents and carers to comment on, and then try out, various scenarios and role plays, comparing successful with less successful interactions. The two children's groups participated in very practical activities around locating feelings in the body, then talking about them and ended with a 'temper tantrum' role play. The teenagers, on the other hand, talked about how to read emotions from facial and other body cues and how communications can so easily be misread and they then tried out effective ways of communicating through role-playing exercises and evaluated their success.

After lunch all the groups came together again and we explained the idea of Family Time. This was adapted from the FBP. The idea of Family Time is conceived of as a weekly fun activity for everyone in the family where the emphasis is on enjoyment, being active together, and not using the time for chores or problem solving. Families struggling to manage life after a bereavement often cannot make having fun together a priority, and the focus may be on getting through the days or weeks individually rather than building in some enjoyable shared activities. We had chosen a collaborative art activity and together families worked on creating a collage entitled 'Our Family' which they could take home with them at the end of the day. This shared activity allowed for discussion as to the kinds of fun activities families could undertake and incorporate into their lives as well as the simple pleasure of sharing in a creative endeavour.

So how successful was this new initiative? Candle has a long tradition of running group days and evenings and this was a radical departure. Many of the parents who came to the Family Workshop are already familiar with our existing groups and found it quite hard to adjust to the change in emphasis from telling individual stories and offering mutual support. Clearly from the feedback we received from parents and carers there was still a need for this sharing of stories to happen but participants welcomed the more didactic approach as well. The children and young people enjoyed the different activities on the whole and participated enthusiastically. They found the role plays easy to engage with and enjoyed the use of humour as well as the hands-on activities. These groups were also much more similar in form and structure to our existing groups and so represented less of a change.

However our groups have always evolved and are always a work in progress and, although this was a significant sidestep, it has allowed us to start to explore a different way of working. We were able to construct a day where adults as well as children and young people, working alongside one another and with one another, could begin to address issues around the very real difficulties of living in a reconfigured family. As one young person wrote after the group:

'I thought it was very helpful … it allowed me to reflect not just on my family but on my life in general'. A parent wrote of the value of looking at how to care for her own wellbeing and of the 'lovely nurturing environment'.

We have another day planned for 2009 and will seek to incorporate both our own evaluations and those from the families who attended into a second Family Workshop day.

Conclusion

In this way a mixed Candle programme of group events has evolved over time, some groups offering a one-off experience of meeting other bereaved children of a similar age and others offering ongoing termly meetings. Within the boundaries of limited time and a restricted budget, this allows different family members a variety of possible ways in which to connect with the project and with other bereaved people.

References

Christ, G.H. (2000) *Healing Children's Grief*. New York: Oxford University Press.

Crossley, D. and Stokes, J. (2002) *Beyond the Rough Rock: Supporting a Child Who has Been Bereaved Through Suicide*. Gloucester: Winston's Wish.

Department for Education and Skills (2004) *Every Child Matters: Change for Children. UK: The Stationary Office*. www.everychildmatters.gov.uk/publications. Accessed 12.01.09.

Dyregrov, A. (2008a) *Grief in Young Children: A Handbook for Adults*. London and Philadelphia: Jessica Kingsley.

Dyregrov, K. and Dyregrov, A. (2008b) *Effective Grief and Bereavement Support: The Role of Family, Friends, Colleagues, Schools and Support Professionals*. London and Philadelphia: Jessica Kingsley.

Foulkes, S.H. (1964) *Therapeutic Group Analysis*. London: Allen and Unwin.

Heegaard, M. (1988) *When Someone Very Special Dies: Children can Learn to Cope With Grief*. Minneapolis USA: Woodland Press.

Kraus, F. and Sinclair, S. *Setting up a Facilitated Self-Help Group: Working with Parents and Carers of Bereaved Children and Young People*. www.childhoodbereavementnetwork. org.uk/documents/settingupafacilitatedselfhelpgroup.pdf accessed 12.01.09.

Kirk, K. and McManus, M. (2002) Containing families' grief; therapeutic group work in a hospice setting. *International Journal of Palliative Nursing,* **8** (10): 470–80.

Lohnes, Kelly L. and Kalter, N. (1994) Preventive intervention groups for parental bereaved children. *American Journal of Orthopsychiatry,* **64** (4): 594–603.

McCarthy, J.R. and Jessup, J. (2005) *Young People, Bereavement and Loss: Disruptive Transitions?* London: National Children's Bureau.

Moreno, J.L. Psychodrama and Psychometry. (1989) *Journal of Group Psychotherapy,* **42** (1).

Pfeffer, C.R. Jiang, H.R., Kakuma, T. et al. (2002) Group intervention for children bereaved by the suicide of a relative. *Journal of American Academy of Child Psychiatry,* **41** (5): 505–13.

Sandler, I.N., Ayers, T.S., and Romer A.L. (2002) Fostering resilience in families in which a parent has died. *Journal of Palliative Medicine,* **5**, 945–56.

Smith, S.C. and Pennells, M. (1995) *Interventions with Bereaved Children.* London: Jessica Kingsley.

Stokes, J. (2004) A Weekend with Winston: bringing people together on a residential group. In Stokes, J.A. *Then, Now and Always: Supporting Children as They Journey Through Grief- A Practitioner's Guide.* Cheltenham: Winston's Wish.

Stroebe, M. and Schut, H. (1999) The dual process model of coping with bereavement: rationale and description. *Death Studies,* **23** (3).

Sunderland, M. (2007) *What every Parent Needs to Know: The Incredible Effects of Love, Nurture and Play on Your Child's Development.* London: Dorling Kindersley.

Yalom, I. Leszcz, M. (2005) *The Theory and Practice of Group Psychotherapy,* 5th edition. New York: Basic books.

Chapter 8

Shrinking the space between people

Di Stubbs

The cornerstone of child bereavement work will always lie in the face to face and person to person connection that is made between practitioner and child or young person. Even though bereavement services for children and their families have grown rapidly in the last fifteen years, we are a long way from the desired situation of every bereaved family having a truly local, open access service on their doorstep. And even if we do one day achieve that, there will always be families for whom individual or group work is not possible or appropriate.

However, almost everyone has access to a telephone, an increasing number of people have access to email and the internet, and many people use text messaging. Creative use of this technology can shrink the space between the practitioner and the bereaved person.

Early intervention

Telephone and email support offer a new twist on the concept of early intervention in bereavement and trauma support. At the end of the line, at a click of a mouse, there can be a highly skilled and experienced practitioner who can make a timely, significant, and lasting difference to bereaved families.

Face to face work

Firstly and briefly for comparison, some characteristics of face to face work with bereaved people include:

- usually an appointment system, often with a considerable waiting list
- within time-restrained hours (e.g. 9 to 5)
- either at the family home, the office of the organization or some other 'clinical' space
- only available in certain parts of the country
- family members become known to the organization
- temptation to 'put on a brave face'

For a bereaved person, exhausted both physically and emotionally, it can be an enormous effort to take the necessary actions to arrive at a face-to-face meeting.

At the end of the line ....

Support over the telephone can have the following characteristics:-

Advantages – for the person making contact

- feeling in control of the communication; the call can be ended at any time with no embarrassment or apology and the caller can even ring off before speaking
- anonymity
- immediacy – calls can be made when there is a need – subject to the helpline's opening hours – without an appointment
- accessibility
- ease of contact – the caller doesn't have to tidy the living room or get dressed
- emotion – for those uncomfortable with expressing emotion, it may be easier to talk without being face to face
- one-way – the caller is the focus of the call.

Disadvantages – for person making contact

- no visual clues on the response coming from the other person – shock, sympathy, etc.
- some people find it harder to communicate and harder to decide whether to trust without seeing the other person.

Advantages – for the person answering

- able to focus on what is being said (and not said) without visual distractions
- can be easier to ask the more difficult questions or explore the more painful areas
- nature of the contact (spontaneity and intimacy) leads to a more quickly established rapport
- the answerer can make notes, look out of the window, or sip a cup of tea without appearing impolite or uninterested.

Disadvantages – for the person answering

- no visual clues that can guide response – is the caller silently struggling ?
- accents can be harder to decipher over the phone.

An intimate disclosure

Some people think that it must feel impersonal talking to a helpline; in practice, most callers find a special intimacy in talking over the phone to someone who makes the time to listen and is felt to care. A caller once described it as 'whispering your pain into someone's ear'.

The quality of the intervention – over the phone as much as in a face-to-face encounter – is determined by the way in which the answerer is able to create for the caller a place that feels safe to share.

The caller has overcome the first barrier to seeking support and guidance by picking up the phone and dialling the number. In a phone communication, tone is what matters most. The right tone transcends accent, class, gender and can make someone stay to talk who was poised to ring off.

If the voice at the end of the line sounds warm without seeming cloying, unhurried without seeming un-bothered, accepting without seeming uncaring, and concerned without seeming intrusive, the caller is more likely to trust it with deep feelings. If the voice is also able to convey a kindly, informed competence and a trustworthy reliability, the relationship between caller and called stands a chance. Most of all, does this voice 'stand alongside' the caller in their pain and confusion and sound as if it will support their choices and actions?

Answering the call

After the caller has decided to trust this voice, the task of relationship is not over. It has to be continually remade throughout the call. This requires a very active form of listening; the answerer must sit up and listen, not sit back. The quality of the listening elicits what the caller wants to say. A helpline answerer has highly privileged access to the caller's thoughts and feelings and has to use this access with great care and consideration.

All good helpline answerers use similar equipment and tools. For example:

- the use of open-ended questions
- reflecting back what the caller has said
- summarizing
- asking what they had thought of doing or saying
- the creative use of 'mmm?'
- 'don't just do something, sit there'
- the therapeutic use of silence.

When providing bereavement support to an adult supporting a bereaved child, a conversation will range over many areas. It may start with listening, emotional support and befriending, move through some information about children and grief, offer some guidance or direct advice, and end with some practical ideas and some more emotional support. It is important that the guidance and information offered is based on experienced practice as well as theory.

A call from a family member is also a call from someone who is experiencing their own bereavement. The child may have lost a parent, a sibling, a grandparent. The caller will have lost a partner, an ex-partner, a child, a parent.

> 'When his Grandfather died, my son said solemnly "I'm a bereaved child" and I thought "so am I"'.

A key element of how a child or young person will respond to the death of someone important is the response of the parent or key carer. Any intervention needs to have a concern for the person in the parental role. Support for them will help secure a better outcome for their family.

The answerer should therefore acknowledge the caller's position before beginning to focus gently on the child. At this point in a helpline call with a bereaved family, the practitioner is conducting a brief assessment of what this death of this person, means to this child, at this time, living in this family and in this community.

The next question the answerer needs to ask him/herself is 'what help/support/ guidance is this family asking me for?'. The subsequent question is 'what do I think this family needs?' It can be quite a temptation to put these two questions the other way around, but it is important to respect and honour the caller's autonomy and start from where they are.

This may now be the time to offer some information, for example, about children's differing developmental understanding of death, about common reactions and responses, about the thoughts and feelings of grief.

After the sharing of information, comes the time for advice or guidance. The intention is to offer any guidance tentatively, always being aware that bereaved people attract well-meaning but infuriating advice as a honey pot attracts bees. The helpline answerer will avoid saying 'if I were you ....' or 'what you need to do now is ....' Instead they will try: 'What have you thought of doing ... ?' 'You may want to consider ....' 'I wonder if you'd thought of ....' 'What would happen if you .....' 'How do you think your child would react if you ....'

The answerer must always keep in mind that this family is operating and needs to operate within their own family context – past, present and future.

The next stage of the helpline call can then be the offering of practical ideas. These are powerful, creative tools and resources to help the family at this time and may include activities and ideas for ways to remember someone who has died.

Other resources can be suggested; books or other printed materials, useful websites, child bereavement services in the caller's locality, or if appropriate the time to explore how the service may be able to offer one-to-one or group support.

The approaching end of the call gives the answerer a chance to summarize, to reflect back, to remind of any key points or actions, and a chance to check that the caller has said all they want to.

It is also the time to encourage the caller to call again, if this is appropriate; to acknowledge their grief and sense of loss; to pay tribute to their care and concern for the children amidst their own grief, and to convey the telephonic equivalent of a warm hand clasp.

After the call

At the end of the call, the answerer needs to reflect on what has been shared and learned, take any necessary actions, follow agreed practices on recording the call and, importantly, seek any support they need for themselves.

Some calls demand every ounce of the answerer's attention, skill, knowledge, and heartstrings. It is essential that the organization has a support mechanism in place for the 'coming down' phase, if required. Debriefing involves the answerer describing the call, any actions to be taken, their own responses, and how they felt they were able to support the caller.

It must not be assumed that a helpline can meet every caller's needs. There will be times when things go less smoothly. All organizations that provide helpline support have to establish policies and procedures that will address challenging issues, and need to provide training and support for helpline answerers.

Outcomes

In offering bereavement support over the phone, it is good to consider what the outcome of a call may be for the caller. A reasonable outcome might be that the concerned adult feels better able, after the call, to support the bereaved child. This, in turn, would mean that the bereaved child or young person is better able to journey through their grief.

Case study

Leo called the helpline, concerned about his 12-year old son, Kip, who had showed no emotion after his mother's death from breast cancer four months earlier. The practitioner explored how Leo was responding himself to his wife's death. Leo explained that he tried to keep things 'bouncing along', didn't mention his wife for fear of upsetting his son, and kept his feelings under strict control until Kip was in bed. The answerer simply and gently asked how Kip might interpret his dad's reactions .... There was an audible moment of realisation.

Leo immediately understood what his responses were telling Kip. As he said 'how can he dare to cry if I don't? How can he talk about her if I never do? I'm going to cry with him tonight'. Twenty minutes had, hopefully, radically changed that family's communication and encouraged the therapeutic sharing of their individual grief.

Calls from children and young people

While having written mainly about receiving calls from adults, it is important to consider briefly calls from young people. Particular training is necessary when preparing to receive calls from children. While, in theory, there may be little or no difference between supporting children or adults who are grieving; in reality, a phone answerer may find themselves becoming involved and affected more quickly and more deeply when talking by phone to a child who is grieving. The use of skills practice ('role play') is very valuable in preparing to answer calls from bereaved young people; better by far to make mistakes on each other.

Discussions about the types of calls that challenge established policies and procedures are important. For example, what if a young caller talks about their drug use or suicide attempts ? What if they tell of a bereaved sibling being physically abused ? What if they have disclosed risk while deliberately with-holding their name or address but have mentioned the name of their school ?

When supporting children over the phone, it is important to be realistic and honest with ourselves as well as with them about the limits of what can be done.

Having said which, the phone offers a tremendous opportunity to engage young people who may feel more confident at speaking – at least initially – to someone they can't see. It also offers a good opportunity to give support at a distance over a longer period by regular, maybe quite short, contacts between the bereaved young person and the practitioner who is working with them.

The Winston's Wish Family Line (08452 030405)

The question of how to reach more families with an early intervention is what prompted Winston's Wish (a community-based child bereavement organiza-tion) to launch the national UK helpline for anyone caring for a bereaved child. By the end of the first eight years (2001 – 2008), over 25,000 people had contacted the service by phone. These people (70% family members, 30% pro-fessionals) in turn, were concerned about around 50,000 bereaved children and young people.

Each call is answered by an experienced and skilled practitioner. That is, the calls are answered by the same person who will also get down on the floor to draw with a six- year old, the same person who will co-ordinate residential groups, the same person who can go alongside an angry adolescent, or despairing parent or guardian. The combination of both a theoretical and experiential basis adds quality to the intervention.

At the click of a mouse ......

For organizations and groups seeking to support bereaved children, young people, and their families, the provision of support through email has to be at least considered since it will be the contact method of choice of much of their target audience.

Advantages – for the person making contact

- control – over content and over ending contact
- anonymity
- immediacy and speed
- accessibility – emails can be sent and replies accessed from anywhere with an internet connection. Email is increasingly used by those with speech and/or hearing difficulties
- privacy
- one way – when a response is wanted but not a conversation
- cost advantage
- normality – most young people and an increasing percentage of the population use email as the communication medium of choice
- written word – it can be easier emotionally and less embarrassing to write rather than to say, there is also the opportunity to review a response before sending it.

Disadvantages – for person making contact

- no clues on the response coming from the other person
- have to wait for response when the emotional need may be urgent
- some people find it harder to put thoughts and feelings into written words.

Advantages – for the person answering

- all content of the communication is available from the outset
- feelings and thoughts – 'you get deeper quicker'
- quality – the response can be improved by checking over each word – and, if required, checking response with someone else before sending
- no struggling with quiet voices, regional accents etc.

- less judgmental – response not clouded by judgments made on clues in the caller's voice
- not distracted by surrounding noise that can affect phone calls
- the response can come from anywhere and anytime with a net connection
- responses to several emails can be prioritized, rather than taking the next call that comes
- the enquirer's email address is known so follow-up can be sensitively offered, if no reply received.

Disadvantages – for answerer

- lack of clues to guide responses, lack of cultural reference points, lack of nuance can make it harder to grasp what is being said
- harder to assess the urgency of the need
- the delay between contact and response cuts the potential for a spontaneous reaction
- harder to convey warmth and empathy through the written word
- it isn't possible to 'use' silence
- harder to pull the conversation round if there is a mistake/misinterpretation and having a written record of response may lead to over-caution.

To e or not to e

Responding to email needs to be seen as an integral part of the service being provided – not an 'add-on'. There are important considerations for a service that intends to communicate with bereaved people by email.

Who will be emailing?

While it is important to be clear about who the primary 'audience' for support is intended to be (so that the service can plan to meet their needs), in practice, whoever it is aimed at, emails will be received from people in other groups (parents, young people, professionals) as well as from the researcher, journalist and the person who has 'come to the wrong shop'. The following points will concentrate mainly on responding to emails from young people.

Who will respond?

Because email is so much part of our world, it may be thought that there is no need for special training in replying. However, it takes real skill and experience to be able to make an assessment of the email writer's needs and feelings – both the stated and unstated – and to respond supportively. Additional training in using the written word therapeutically is required; while the medium allows the possibility of consultation on a response that is not possible with a phone call or face-to-face work.

It might be assumed that email support is best handled by younger people. In practice, older people may be more comfortable and familiar with responding using the written word (emailing is equivalent to writing a letter).

The tone is just as important as in a helpline or face-to-face contact. In responding to a young person, the tone needs to convey an impression of a person who can be supportive of all thoughts and feelings, has helpful information but is not going to lecture, and is fundamentally on your side.

The response

In practice, emails can be answered at a remote location at a convenient time. If answerers are working off-site it is important to have support structures in place.

The usual response time needs to be advertised and adhered to. In practice, writers seem to accept a 24-hour turn-around.

While the medium allows for a long detailed response, in practice there is a balance to be set between providing enough information and support and keeping the reply within a reasonable length. The temptation to demonstrate erudition needs to be tempered by realising how intimidating this can be for the recipient.

Recognizing the language

Email uses a vibrant, direct, and immediate language that is suited to the communication of feelings and thoughts. It is unlikely that an email message from a young person will be correctly spelt or grammatical, but it will be powerful.

> My dad died nearly a yer ago.And scince then my life feel rubish.and i somtimes just want to die. When will i stop like this?

> it is my mum who has died she died of a brain hemeridge it was all sudden. i live with my dad i have no brothers or sisters i am 12 years off age my bday is today

In replying to an email from a young person, it is not necessary to use the same language – for example, to deliberately mis-spell a word to seem 'cool' and 'in touch'; but it is necessary to be direct, non-fussy and non-academic.

Policies, practices, and procedures

Email response should be in integral part of any service, subject to the same policies, practices and procedures as face-to-face or group work. In addition to those mentioned before, these need to include a policy on data protection, record keeping and storage.

Policies may need to be re-considered in the light of email support. Here are some questions:

- How can you enact your child protection policy if you do not know the child's location ?
- How do you support a suicidal young person when you do not know their location ?
- To what extent are you prepared to attempt to trace someone ?
- How mindful do you need to be to the possibility of someone else reading your response ?
- If you are offering advice that can be printed out and kept, do you need to have indemnity insurance ?
- For how long will you keep records ? And will you keep these electronically or on paper ?
- How do you ensure continuity if your service starts an email 'conversation' with someone?

What makes email support particularly appropriate for young people who have been bereaved ?

Many young people can find it hard to seek support from a stranger face-to-face. Even with those close to them they may struggle to reach a point of easy communication about thoughts and feelings of grief.

It is much easier to tap out a question or a comment while already sitting at the computer doing something else. Sending it off doesn't involve a major commitment to a relationship with the person or organization to which it is sent. The communication takes place at a distance yet it feels like an intimate connection. When a reply comes, there is no pressure to respond in turn. The emailer can feel and act diffidently, crudely, angrily, and no-one gets hurt. It is about the nearest one can get to a safe expression of grief.

The medium has all the advantages outlined above – immediate, convenient, tentative, fleeting – that makes it suit a young person who is unsure about seeking support following bereavement.

The future for email

Email support will become an important part of every child bereavement service. Through email, bereaved young people whom services may struggle to reach in more traditional ways can be contacted and offered a warm, human response to their grief.

Using the web to reach young people

One of the real challenges for a child bereavement service is to engage children, young people, and their parents by finding a variety of communications that will work for all ages. For those with access to the Internet, it is now usually the first choice for those seeking to understand more about a subject or seek support.

A website is, nowadays, a necessary requirement for any organization seeking to have a public profile; but it can also become so much more than simply a promotion of the organization's existence. For a child bereavement service, one strong reason to have a website is as a means of engaging bereaved young people. Additionally, information and guidance on supporting bereaved children and young people can be put into the public domain where parents and carers, professionals and, in particular, schools can instantly access and use it.

The young person's perspective

You can imagine a bereaved teenager, sitting at the computer in their room or even at school – feeling very diffident, very suspicious, very reluctant – and steeling themselves to search for information on bereavement. It is quick and easy to click away from a website about bereavement and onto something more enticing.

Therefore the tone of any website (or youth pages with an organization's website) need to convey the qualities of the service, for example, that this service is approachable, trustworthy, and accepting of people's feelings and thoughts. There is, of course, no control that says only young people will access pages aimed at young people; equally it can be assumed that young people will explore throughout the site and need to feel acknowledged and respected wherever they go.

Pages aimed at young people – like all good website content – need to be accessible to those with impaired sight or hearing and to young people with low literacy levels or for whom English is not their first language.

Web-based services, including message boards and other interactive activities, have many potential advantages for bereaved young people providing:

- anonymity
- privacy
- ease of access
- immediacy
- accessibility – to all regardless of physical ability, race, culture, gender – and no need to travel
- availability – 24-7
- one-to-machine – no obvious contact with another person
- freedom of expression
- culturally relevant – meeting young people on their own 'ground'.

Logging out

'Actually, I don't like to admit it, but I felt a bit better afterwards'.
'I talked to mum about dad for the first time since he died'.
'I'll have a look tomorrow to see if anyone else feels like me'.

The web has transformed communication between people, but it's not a magic answer in itself. The development of a website does not remove the need to develop and deliver other direct services for bereaved teenagers.

www.winstonswish.org.uk

Like most organizations, the Winston's Wish website provides a window to the range of services available and carries a wealth of information for parents, carers and professionals, especially schools, on how to support bereaved children. A large interactive section within the website is specifically aimed at young people.

Through this area of the site, bereaved young people are able to engage in a range of activities around remembering the person who has died and expressing feelings and thoughts of grief; these include a starscape of memories, grafitti wall and podcasts. They can gain access to information about death, dying, and bereavement. Young people can also communicate with us by asking a specific question by email or with one another through often moving and powerful messages on the moderated message boards.

HRU? RUOK? *(How are you? Are you OK?)*

Another possibility to add to the opportunities to reach bereaved people is the use of text messaging: a technology that has almost universal acceptance amongst young people.

Responding to text messages should be an integral part of the overall package of services offered. In place there need to be training, adapted policies, procedures, quality control, monitoring, etc. The points made above relating to responding to emails are equally relevant here.

Texting has the advantages of email to young people (please see the longer list above). In summary these are:

- immediacy and speed
- anonymity
- control
- accessibility
- culturally-relevant and normal
- low cost.

Text messaging can be used to support bereaved young people in the following ways:

- a message on an important day – anniversary of the death, birthday of the person who has died etc

- a gentle 'thinking of you' message when they are going through a rough time

- an encouraging reminder of the next appointment or group meeting

- a follow-up to an individual session – 'good to see you today'

- a continuing conversation with a caller – albeit one conducted in short bursts (software exists to make this possible)

- a first point of contact for someone exploring the service. ('Text INFO to 07979 xxxx'). The response could start a supportive connection for the young person.

Conclusion

It could be said that the provision of emotional support is at its purest between two people – one who needs support and one who cares to give it – irrespective of their ages, genders, nationalities, and even location. This chapter has looked at how technology can be used to provide relevant services to bereaved young people, their families and the professionals who care for them.

For many adults, a helpline call, an email, or the opportunity to read through a web page will be sufficient to enable them to continue to support their bereaved children. For some, the call, mail, or page will point them to fresh ideas, new insights and useful resources. For a few, the technology will act as a gateway to the services available nationally and locally. For young people, emails, texts and websites may be the most bearable way to make the first tentative approach for help and support.

The technology is succeeding in shrinking the space between people.

Chapter 9

Loss for children with learning disability

Linda McEnhill

The face of children's bereavement care has changed beyond recognition in the last decade. As a result of pioneering practitioners and organizations such as the Childhood Bereavement Network, the profile of bereaved children has been raised and services specifically designed and funded to meet their needs. Of course there is still much to be done. Funding and services remain patchy and the public is not yet fully cognisant of the needs of bereaved children, but the revolution has begun. Sadly not so for children with learning disabilities (LD), many of whom experience bereavement (of peers at least) more often and whose needs may be more complex but remain largely unmet even by the leading services and thinkers in the field.

Current conceptualizations of 'resilience', which are properly influencing emerging bereavement service models, are a case in point. Whilst it is clear that we have well established notions of 'vulnerability' in people with disabilities, it is not so clear that we have any concept of what resilience might look like in such people and especially in children with LD. This chapter will begin by defining what a learning disability 'is' and clarifiying what it 'is not', specifically in relation to bereavement. The chapter will then explore issues related to disability and bereavement and consider how to help children with LD enhance their sense of personal identity and their consequent ability to manage the crisis of bereavement.

Definitions of learning disability

The World Health Organization (1992) has defined learning disability as *a state of arrested or incomplete development of mind.*

Whilst there are numerous definitions of LD they normally include elements of 'social dysfunction' (centring on communication or daily living skills) alongside cognitive impairment (often measured in terms of IQ levels), which are irreversible and began in childhood.

The causes of LD are as diverse as the types of LD, involving pre and post-birth conditions or trauma. Sometimes the LD is accompanied by physical impairments or autistic spectrum disorders (ASD). The latter, whilst not affecting intellectual ability, may have a significant impact on the experience and expression of emotions including attachment and loss.

LD certainly increases the complexity of assessing which services to offer. It is important however to consider some of the things which a LD does not constitute.

- It does not constitute, in itself, the inability to bond, form meaningful relationships and to experience their absence as distressing loss. We know from the work of child psychologists that children as young as seven months of age experience separation anxiety (Seigler 2006). Very few children with LD, no matter how severe their disability, operate below this level. Therefore we would expect that children with LD will experience absence as loss and the breaking of attachments as distressing as children generally do, though the expression of this may be harder to interpret.

- Necessarily impaired emotional intelligence. Sinason (1992) demonstrated that there could be 'emotional intelligence left intact and rich regardless of how crippled performance intelligence was'.

- The inability to change, develop or grow. All children learn from experience and can therefore benefit from sharing the 'normalizing' grief experiences of others.

- Necessarily complex grief. There is no reason to suggest that children simply by virtue of their disability will experience unresolved grief, any more than there is reason to suggest they will not experience grief at all.

- The inability to retain healthy 'continuing bonds' with the deceased. Studies of adults with LD have shown that they continued to dream of their deceased loved ones some 20 years after their death (Turner and Graffam 1987). The evidence suggests that such remembering was internally generated and not stimulated or supported by individuals external to the bereaved person.

Disability and bereavement

For families where the bereaved child has a LD there are some issues which require special consideration in the assessment and facilitation of bereavement. These include: attachment, cognition, communication, and elements of resilience related to personal identity.

Attachment

Blackman's work (2003) on bereavement and LD reminds us of the importance of the concept of attachment as previously developed by Bowlby and others.

In terms of the child with LD there are a number of challenges to the development of a secure attachment initiated either by the circumstances of the birth, the knowledge of the disability, family reaction, or any combination of these. If we consider the newborn child with LD, a number of circumstances may come into play including:

- Trauma of birth (the mother and child may be physically ill after the birth)
- Difficulties with feeding
- Emotional/physical robustness of the parents (this is likely to be influenced by whether the 'disability' was expected, family values, and norms concerning disability, guilt, blame etc.)
- Separation due to birth complications
- Continuous separations in early childhood due to hospital stays which may result in bonding issues with siblings and parents
- The child may lack behaviours which attract the parents' attention and thereby 'disconnect' or fail to establish bond enhancing behaviours. This may be a particular issue for children with ASD and may be exacerbated by the fact that children with this disorder may not like being held or cuddled (Ryaskin 2004)
- Parents may 'over protect' the child.

Parkes (1991) has demonstrated the link between attachment types and complexity of grief. In a family where the child has a disability, this may be one of the elements which influences both how the child is expected to grieve, and how the child actually does. Insecure and ambivalent attachments are often intensified by service responses.

Cognition

It is important to remember that adapting normal interventions to the developmental level of the child is relatively straightforward. The caveat to this is where there is significant dissonance between the chronological age and developmental stage of the child. Children in this situation should be offered 'age appropriate' interventions which have been adapted to their developmental stage. This need not be complicated as is demonstrated by the response of one 'open access' service.

This particular child bereavement service offers a number of group programmes each year to children within its geographical area. Individual and family assessments are carried out in advance of a place being offered on the programme, including specific needs of the child as a result of disability or the loss experience. The service routinely has one or two children with LD, or other special needs, within its chronological peer groups.

In groups including children with LD, an extra worker, who is briefed regarding specific issues related to disability or environment, is assigned. Where the child is able to 'cope' independently, or the group successfully adapts to meet the needs of the child, the extra leader works with the whole group. Where the child requires additional assistance the worker can support on a one to one basis. Thus the child's life experience is respected and their cognitive needs, where necessary, are met within the group. This is important otherwise an older child with a LD might find themselves in the same group as a younger sibling and this might impede their expression of grief, or impact on their sense of identity within the family.

Specific cognitive issues vary according to the individual child, the particular LD and the child's life experience but the following issues should be considered:

- Conceptualization: the child may not link concepts as expected and therefore although they knew their parent was ill, may not have expected the death

- Developmental stage: the child may be at an earlier developmental stage than their age would suggest and this may influence the sense that they have made of the death

- Death concept: Some children with LD may take longer to fully understand the significance of the death and may initially therefore appear untroubled, if not somewhat excited, by all the comings and goings initiated by the event. Even mature children with LD may have difficulty understanding the concept of time and this can also impede their comprehension of the death

- Misunderstandings: though possible with all children, they are often increased in children with LD because people do not check out what the child says for fear of drawing attention to the LD. It is possible that a child can be using language in one way (e.g. daddy's gone to heaven) whilst understanding it quite differently (as in the concept of hell) and for this to go unchecked for some time

- Children with LD may teach themselves through experience (which may include the physical 'acting out' of situations which are difficult to understand). Children with LD are as resourceful as their peers and will often find innovative ways of explaining the death to themselves.

Communication

Many children with LD use and understand speech, others don't use speech but do understand it. With this majority, we can use much of what we already do as long as we remember to keep it concrete and at the appropriate developmental level. Those children who do not use speech can, and should be included, though help may need to be sought from family members or other skilled professionals to enable understanding of their communication and the impact the intervention is having upon them. Partnerships with local special needs schools are invaluable as staff will be expert communicators, but may not understand the complexity of grief experienced or how to facilitate its resolution.

There are few written resources to consult but Sanderson (1995) helpfully reminds us that much communication will be behavioural. *If they feel safe, bereaved children will tell us how they feel. The most profoundly disabled will show us.* Of course this does not tell us how to understand what the behaviour is communicating. Oswin (1984) has looked at 'separation anxiety' behaviours and found a high correlation with the behaviour of bereaved people with LD. She suggests that the following behaviours are indicative of grief:

- Searching (very physical, including rummaging or digging in earth)
- Bewilderment (e.g. wandering, twirling curtains)
- Comfort seeking (needing close physical contact)
- Reassurance seeking (e.g. constant questioning)
- Protest (arguing, fighting)
- Mourning (e.g. crying and rocking behaviours).

The practitioner (in both individual and group sessions) needs to develop an awareness of the verbal and non-verbal behaviours of individuals with LD as these are likely to be good indicators of how the child is being affected by the work. As previously suggested, some children with LD will employ behaviour to enable them to understand complex concepts, almost like 'method acting'. Some of the more creative therapies can facilitate this, for example sand tray work or dramatherapy.

Identity and grief work

It has been suggested that enhancing one's sense of personal identity, enhances one's ability to deal with crisis and change. With children support can be as simple as Life Story work (Ryan and Walker 1985, McEnhill 1993).

It is important to consider how disability affects the child's sense of personal identity and this current loss. This includes how a child with a LD conceive of themselves and the nature of their earliest formative memories. Whether the bereaved child is taking part in a group or individual work, areas which may be helpfully explored include:

- Whether the birth was a celebration/sadness – Many parents report not receiving congratulations cards or gifts for their newborn because friends and family did not know how to respond to the disability. Sinason (1992) suggests that implicitly and explicitly people with LD experience society's 'death wish' towards them as a feeling from the outset that their existence is unacceptable. It is easier for children in this situation to believe they are the cause of their parent's hardship and ultimate death

- Models of dealing with disability – Todd (2003) suggests that much support offered to parents on the news of disability conforms to a bereavement counselling model which, whilst well intentioned, entrenches the view that children with disabilities lead 'tragic lives' and that their deaths, when they occur, are consequently a 'blessed release'

- Messages about role in family – Irrespective of actual 'place' in the family hierarchy the role attributed is often of a younger child or focuses on dependency. This can result in the disabled child/adult being left out of information or rituals concerning the illness or death

- Similarities or differences – Very often children with LD are assumed to be more like their LD peers than their biological family members, this is especially so if the child has a syndrome which makes him instantly recognisable as having the condition. This can lead to a sense of alienation and a lack of understanding of the emotional needs of the child

- Ability or disability – The need to provide educational support or services overtly focuses on the child's disabilities rather than abilities and can feed an assumption that the child will not have the internal resources to deal with bereavement

- Passive or active attributes – Children with LD may be 'over socialized' into passivity and inhibition of active expressions of emotion, resulting in defensive 'secondary handicaps' which will need to be overcome before any real grief work can be undertaken (Sinason 1992)

- Recognizing/valuing relationships – The identification of people with LD as somehow 'other' can result in their emotional attachments not being taken seriously and their losses remaining unacknowledged even when of close family members. Hollins (2003) reported that 47% of adults with LD did not attend their parents' funerals

- The unknown – People with disabilities experience much higher levels of abuse than the general public. The trusted bereavement helper may become the confidant of this 'secret'

- Remembering – Children with LD may need help to structure their memories, to have anniversaries recorded, and to have the uniqueness of their relationship with the deceased treasured.

The aim of the bereavement worker is to come alongside the child, to hear their story and by doing so, and by reframing elements appropriately, to extend the child's understanding of themselves, their world and their loss. Some of this work is profoundly painful and workers need to prepare themselves for the strong feelings that the cumulative losses of people with disabilities can engender. It may be worth remembering that this bereavement offers the child with LD an uncommon opportunity to explore their internal world and to enhance their ability to deal with loss.

Sadly most of the 'resilience' literature, as it relates to children, has not yet included disability within its dialogue. Many of the check lists of factors that promote resilience have little relevance to children with LD or the measurement of their resilience. Serious attention needs to be given to whether the current models hold when scrutinized from a disability perspective. As Monroe and Oliviere (2007) point out, we should not be thinking of resilient populations (and conversely 'vulnerable' groups) but of individuals and their 'multiple paths to resilience'. Thus although it has been suggested that 'cognitive ability is a strong and constant predictor of resilience in childhood and adolescence' (Stokes 2007), this needs to be explored more fully taking into account the lived experiences of individuals with disabilities. As professionals we have to avoid seeing the world only through the eyes of the services that we manage. Most people (with disabilities or not) are resilient enough not to need or desire our interventions and we are therefore always (even in open access services) researching within a sub-group which may not be wholly representative of the general population.

Children with LD are certainly capable of resilience in bereavement, often against much higher odds and losses than the 'ordinary' child experiences. Sinason (1992) emphasizes these added difficulties, saying of adults and children with LD that they are:

> '... still too rarely seen to have words and thoughts of value inside them and only too rarely provided with a means of interpreting them or having them interpreted. It is not surprising that they can give up the exhausting and unequal struggle for communication and keep their thoughts locked up in their heads forever. However unlike diaries or poems or books that are hidden away, thoughts unformed and unspoken become a store house of pain'.

We must find better ways to engage with children with LD and to enable them to teach us how to be resilient and resourceful in our approaches to supporting them in bereavement.

References

Blackman, N. (2003) *Loss and Learning Disability*. London: Worth Publishing.

Hollins, S., Raji, O. and Drinnan, A. (2003) How far are people with learning disabilities involved in funeral rites? *British Journal of Learning Disability*, 31(1): 42–45.

McEnhill, L. (1993) Unpublished MSW dissertation. *Bereavement and People With Learning Difficulties: A Pilot Study in the Use of Life Story Books as a Counselling Method.* University of Dundee.

Monroe B. and Oliviere D. (2007) *Resilience in Palliative Care: achievement in adversity.* Oxford: Oxford University Press.

Oswin, M. (1984) *They Keep Going Away: A Critical Study of Short-Term Residential Care Services for Children Who are Mentally Handicapped.* London: King Edward's Hospital Fund for London.

Parkes, C.M. (1991) Attachment, bonding and psychiatric problems after bereavement in adult life. In: Parkes, C.M., Hinde, J.S., Marris, P. *Attachment Across the Life Cycle.* England: Routledge. p. 268–292.

Ryan, Walker R. (1985) *Making Life Story Books.* London: BAAF.

Ryaskin, O.T. (2004) *Trends in Autism Research.* New York: Nova Science Publishers.

Sanderson, J. (1995) Helping families and professionals to work with children who have learning difficulties. In Smith, S.C. and Pennells, M. (eds) *Interventions with Bereaved Children.* London: Jessica Kingsley Publishers. pp. 210–231.

Siegler, R (2006) *How Children Develop: Exploring Child Development.* New York: Worth Publishers.

Sinason, V. (1992) *Mental Handicap and the Human Condition: New Approaches From the Tavistock.* London: Free Association Books.

Stokes, J. (2007) Resilience and bereaved children: helping a child to develop a resilient mind-set following the death of a parent. In Monroe, B. and Oliviere, D. (eds) *'Resilience in Palliative Care: Achievement in Adversity'.* Oxford: Oxford University Press. pp 39–66.

Todd, S. (2003) Death does not become us: the absence of death and dying in intellectual disability research. *Journal of Gerontological Social Work,* **38**(1): 225–239.

Turner, J.L. and Graffam, J.H. (1987) Deceased loved ones in the dreams of mentally retarded adults. *American Journal of Mental Retardation,* **92**: 282–289.

World Health Organisation (1992) The ICD: 10 classification of mental and behavioural disorders: Clinical descriptions and diagnostic guidelines. Geneva.

Chapter 10

Co-creating memory: supporting very young children

Patsy Way

Chapter 7 describes Jermain's experience with his father in a group context in co-creating memories of his mother after she had died in a road traffic crash. At three years old, some would argue that Jermain was too young to remember much about his mother or understand the implications of her death.

Following Piagetian (1963) thinking on children's development, it is argued that children's abilities to understand and remember early experiences rely on cognitive understandings (Kenyon 2001). Rolls et al, (2004 p301) argue that research on children has often been conducted in a positivist frame of scientific method, using methods that privilege observation of children as passive objects. Attention is given to what happens to them and the processes they undergo, rather than to what they do or say. In this model of thinking, memory would be viewed solely as a retrieval process.

Memory of event → thought recreated in the brain → retrieved at a later date and verbalized

Viewed in this way, young children are not very successful in recalling early events. Asked to give a coherent account of a series of events out of context and without prompts, many three year olds could not describe memories of someone who has died. However, recent research suggests that young children may remember more than previously thought (Schaffhausen 2000). To her mother's amazement, Silverman (2002 p2) vividly recalled her grandfather's death when she was only two years old. Nevertheless, many young bereaved children will not be able to access memories with Silverman's clarity. Many children have few or no memories and fear losing those they have. Georgina, aged five, for example, told her mother, 'It's like I don't know daddy any more and I can't think of his voice'.

Madigan (1997 p339) says that he was consistently taught that his memories were personal to him and his responsibility. If one forgets something, one should think 'harder' in order to remember. For some practical purposes, such as locating lost car keys, individual accountability and reliance on accurate memory of a location will be important. However, Sampson (1993 p121) argues for a different view of memory: 'we are not calling up a trace laid down somewhere in our inner computer banks: rather we are engaged in a process of constructing an event in a current situation'. From this position, memories are seen as jointly constructed in joint conversation. This echoes Walter (1999 p82), 'the dead live on in conversation among the living'. What I describe as co-remembering practices appear to be very current in bereavement literature relating to adults (Neimeyer 2001 Walter 1999 Klass et al. 1996). This may be a useful frame in which to view the remembering abilities of very young children.

In telling family stories, we are inevitably very selective from memory. Leroy (Chapter 7) had explained to Jermain that his mother had had a road traffic crash, had been rushed to hospital in an ambulance and the doctors and nurses had tried very hard to save her but had been unable to, so she went to heaven. Leroy had made a brave attempt at an explanation in the face of family members who argued that such efforts were futile at best and damaging at worst. Jermain had, as children do, accepted this explanation and understood the non-verbal message that further questioning was not welcome.

When we revisited the subject together, his questions revealed the extent of the thought he had given to his mother's death. He was confused that his mother, who loved him so much, seemed to have made no effort to return from heaven to visit him. Was she alright or in pain from the accident? Was she missing them? Was heaven a good place for her?[1] As one might predict (Christ 2000 p46–70), such concerns were accompanied by very clingy behaviours when Leroy tried to leave Jermain at preschool or with other carers, and this in turn was challenging Leroy's ideas about his own competence as a parent.

We talked and played out events leading up to his mother's death and the funeral and discussed what people might mean by heaven. His mother loved him and would want to visit him but her body no longer worked. His father's active participation in this process enabled him to see that his ongoing questions and ideas were welcomed and respected.

For Jermain this was the beginning of a process. He continued for a few months to ask his father when his mother would return, but as he talked about her his account of what had happened and how she had died became more coherent and consistent. Tummy aches and clingy behaviour subsided in the following months as Leroy put secure routines in place for eating and bedtimes

---

[1] Lansdown et al. (1997) questioned children about their views of an afterlife. Answers suggested they did not necessarily think heaven a good place. 'Heaven' is not in itself an explanation of where or how someone is after death.

and Jermain regained confidence in the consistent elements in his life and routines.

As demonstrated in a Leeds Animation Workshop DVD (2002), very young children are capable of very strong and immediate emotional reactions to the death of someone important to them, even though they are not able to verbalize or give an account of their feelings. It would seem that most young children have not yet developed the complex neocortical networks necessary for this. Dyregrov (2008 p45–65) argues for the importance of keeping children in contact with concrete memories, such as a favourite object or item of clothing linked to the dead person. He discusses ways in which participation in rituals can help children's understanding and sense of inclusion in an important family event. He shows the importance of play in making sense of events for the child in a changing world.

Children demonstrate knowledge and understanding in many ways, not necessarily verbal. Drama, story-telling and other creative means can reveal the depth of a child's understanding of context.

Case study

Charise, aged four, talked to a teaching assistant at school in a very direct way about her older sister Tamsin who 'got dead' after being in hospital for a long time, 'and now she's a star'. She appeared to the assistant to have understood that her sister could not return. However, to her distraught mother she would say comforting things such as 'she will come back for Christmas' which would further distress her parents and confirm to them that 'she's just so confused, she doesn't understand'. However, it is interesting that Charise was entirely consistent in speaking differently about her sister at home and at school. Her responses could be understood as very sophisticated, using different modes of thinking in different contexts. She was deeply aware of her mother's desperate sorrow and responded with loving reassurance. With professionals in school, she gave a different account of her story, as she understood it. If she had been asked, out of context, if her sister would come home or not and be as she was before, the response would probably be 'don't know' as Charise would not have a context in which to pick up cues and expectations.

Neimeyer (2001) argues that meaning reconstruction in response to loss is the central process involved in grieving. He argues this is a social as well as a cognititve practice. Christ (2000 p47) observed that children 'benefited greatly by being able to talk about the dead person at home after they participated in bereavement groups. One mother speculated that her child probably learned a vocabulary in the group that facilitated this expression'.

Beyond trying to make ordered sense of one's experience, is there value in playing out, storying, and co-creating memories? The evidence from the narrative analyses of Main and colleagues (1997) suggest that, for healthy attachments to occur, the coherence of one's story and the way one has managed to process difficult events appears to be more critical than the severity of trauma involved in the events themselves.

From this one might assume that, at a critical time of change and disorganization for a family following bereavement, it is very important to support the youngest members, along with the whole family, in constructing narratives that make sense and integrate lived experience. This involves supporting them in understanding and storying what has happened and connecting them to their own strengths and resources and those in the family and wider system. It seems crucial to include parents and carers in this process since they carry the memories for the children and will be in a position to continue co-remembering as children grow. If they are supported initially and feel comfortable to talk directly and simply to their children about someone who has died, they are more likely to continue the process as children get older and expand their questions and curiosities about the person who died.

Gemma (8) and Stephen (6) demonstrated the supportive effects of this kind of help from a parent. I met them four years after their mother had died when their father brought them to the Candle playroom. Had their father not spoken to me earlier, I would have been totally astounded by what followed.

Case study

Gemma launched immediately into her story. 'Well, I remember when I was born and daddy drove mummy and me back from the hospital. I was wearing the yellow babygrow nanny gave me. Mummy lay on the settee and she had big trousers on because her tummy was still big from having me. Mummy and daddy took turns holding me and taking pictures'. She produced the relevant photographs and her younger brother managed to interrupt her enthusiastic flow to tell me of his memories of his first birthday, including details about the cake mummy had made.

These children had been supported in co-remembering by their remarkable parents who began recording memories before the children were born and before their mother had received a terminal diagnosis of cancer. They did not want the only and dominant memories to be of her death (reminiscent of Stokes' work with dying mothers 2008). The children were actively encouraged to co-remember events from their birth onwards. They understood she was ill, visited her in hospital, and were included in funeral rituals and memorial events, but these events are part of a wider story about a mother who loved and cared for them. Very early important memories were scaffolded for them using video, photos, story, and play to rehearse over again the crucial part she played in their early life. Perhaps, like Silverman, they do have some mental images of very early experiences or perhaps they are entirely co-remembered. For practical purposes this does not really matter.

I have argued that children need support to make sense of the experience of bereavement, even when they have little or no memories as conventionally understood. I suggest this is important for developing a coherent self-narrative, and for forming secure attachments in the future. Memory is complex and young children need help to co-remember someone important in their past and into their future. Adults can actively engage with this through play and age-appropriate talk and support young children's growing sense of identity.

References

Christ, G. (2000) *Healing Children's Grief: Surviving a Parent's Death From Cancer*. Oxford: Oxford University Press.

Dyregrov, A. (2008) *Effective Grief and Bereavement Support: The Role of Family, Friends, Colleagues, Schools and Support Professionals*. London and Philadelphia: Jessica Kingsley.

Kenyon, B.L. (2001) Current research in children's conceptions of death: a critical review. *Omega Journal of Death and Dying*, **43** (1).

Klass, D., Silverman, S. and Nickerman, S. (eds) (1996) *Continuing Bonds: New Understandings of Grief*. Washington DC: Taylor and Francis.

Lansdown, R., Jordan, N., and Frangoulis, S. (1997) Children's concept of an afterlife. *Bereavement Care*, **14** (2): 16–18.

Leeds Animation workshop (2002) Not too young to grieve (DVD/VHS) Leeds.

Neimeyer, R. (2001) *Meaning Reconstruction and the Experience of Loss*. Washington DC: American Psychological Association.

Main, M. (1997) Metacognitive knowledge, metacognitive monitoring and singular (coherent) vs multiple (incoherent) models of attachment. Findings and directions for future research. In Parkes, C.M., Stevenson-Hinde, J. and Marris, P. *Attachment Across the Life Cycle*. London: Routledge.

Madigan, S. (1997) Re-considering memory: remembering lost identities back toward remembered selves. In Smith, C. and Nylund, D. (eds) *Narrative Therapies With Children and Adolescents*. New York and London: Guildford Press.

Piaget, J. (1954) *The Construction of Reality in the Child*. New York: Basic Books.

Rolls, L. and Payne, S. (2004) Childhood bereavement services: issues in UK service provision. *Mortality*, **9** (4).

Sampson, E. (1993) *Celebrating the Other: A Dialogic Account of Human Nature*. Boulder, CO: Westview Press.

Schaffhausen, J. (2000) *Gone But Not Forgotten? The Mystery Behind Infant Memories*. www.brainconnection.com/topics/?main=fa/Infantile-amnesia (accessed 16.11.05).

Silverman, P.H. (2000) *Never Too Young to Know: Death in Children's Lives*. New York: Oxford University Press.

Stokes, J. *Mummy Diaries*. www.channel4.com/mummydieries Accessed 18.010.09.

Walter, T. (1999) *On Bereavement*. Buckingham: Open University Press.

Chapter 11

The extended warranty

Frances Kraus

The title of this book was chosen to reflect the reality of work with bereaved children and families. Professionals and volunteers in the field are aware that for many bereaved families, a brief intervention will be the only one possible. The reasons are varied, sometimes arising from families' difficulties in making the commitment to attending sessions on a long term basis or from a need to ration scarce resources, but this does not mean that a short term intervention is not also an appropriate therapeutic choice.

The St Christopher's Candle Project was established in 1998, and offers short term bereavement focused intervention to children, young people, and families bereaved by death in South East London. We cover five London boroughs, with a total population of about 1.2 million. The boroughs are a mixture of the inner city and suburbs, and are very ethnically and socially diverse. Most [80%] of the Candle families come from areas that score highly on the Index of Multiple Deprivation, and 45% of the children we see are from an ethnic background that is not white British. Many (65%) of the referrals to Candle are for children who have experienced a sudden and traumatic death.

Agencies have their own reasons for choosing to deliver a brief intervention, which may be pragmatic or therapeutic. Children's bereavement projects are still a scarce resource in most parts of the UK, (see Chapter 1) and any resource that offers free counselling for children will be rapidly over-subscribed. Funders of services want to see evidence of outputs and outcomes, and in a field where appropriate outcome measures have to date not yet been developed, outputs, often quantified as numbers of children seen or groups delivered, become more important. The Candle Project has a staff team consisting of 3.3 full time equivalent workers including a part time administrator, plus a sessional worker, and a team of volunteers who help with the groups. Candle attempts to avoid long waiting times for families, recognizing that a long wait is counter-therapeutic for a child ready for bereavement counselling. Working short term helps to restrict waiting times, as staff caseloads are not full with long term clients.

Our experience in the Candle Project validates a positive view of the therapeutic value of a brief intervention. The service was developed using the experience of a short term intervention that had worked well previously in a consultancy service offered by St Christopher's Hospice (Monroe 1997). This service was evaluated at the time, and had confirmed our belief that if help was delivered swiftly when the families were most receptive, short term work was appropriate for the majority of bereaved children.

Bereavement is a normal process of adjustment to a major life event, and attending counselling sessions long term can reduce a family's coping skills by creating a dependency on the bereavement counsellor or agency. Children form attachments very quickly, and the ending of a long term counselling relationship can give them another loss to deal with.

In common with other agencies in the bereavement field, Candle has had to engage with the challenges of providing a short term intervention. Bereaved families encounter many difficulties managing the practical issues that arise and at the same time trying to find space and time to grieve. These issues make their lives more complex and demanding and make it hard for them to attend appointments consistently. However short the intervention, school, work and home demands are more immediate and pressing, and commitment to counselling sometimes comes low down on their day to day priorities. Project staff need to be able to create an effective working alliance very quickly, and build on it to overcome the inevitable disruptions that will arise as families fail to make appointments due to illness, accidents or forgetfulness.

For some families, pre-existing problems necessitate referral to other agencies either before or following intervention and, in this case, we discuss this initially with the referrer. The project sometimes receives referrals where bereavement, though a factor in a child's life, is not the most important or most pressing issue.

Case study

A young man whose grandmother had died was refusing to leave his room and becoming very verbally aggressive to his single parent mother, who referred him to Candle. After meeting with her, it was clear to the worker that his problems were long standing and needed a mental health assessment, so the family doctor was contacted to arrange this.

Sometimes children may need an assessment for Post Traumatic Stress Disorder before bereavement work is started. This necessitates a referral to a Child and Adolescent Mental Health team or a Traumatic Stress clinic. (Chapter 16)

Many families, however, may face issues that arise as a result of the bereavement, after the counselling has ended. In this chapter, I examine the idea of the extended warranty, a term borrowed from the insurance field where it is used to mean an extension of the usual term of guarantee for a new purchase. In our setting it is a response to the problems and issues that may arise for a bereaved family by offering them the opportunity for further limited contact if needed. Approximately 15% of our referrals every year are from families we have worked with previously, who are asking for further involvement.

How is the intervention structured?

The service begins with the first contact. Many children are referred by their parent or carer, and whatever the referral source, the initial contact by project staff is by telephone, which provides an opportunity to begin the assessment process (Stokes 2004) and to deliver an immediate intervention relevant to the family. Parents are often very anxious when they first phone us, and value the reassurance and support in that first call, which may be quite lengthy. Telephone intervention is discussed in more detail in Chapter 8. Candle takes over 450 calls every year from parents and professionals. Many of these calls do not result in a referral, for a variety of reasons. Some are out of our area and need referral on, others are training requests, and some are from parents or professionals who need to be able to talk though things with an 'expert', and having done that are reassured and do not need further involvement from Candle at the time (Levy 2004).

When the referral form comes in, an acknowledgement is sent out to parent and referrer, if appropriate. When the project is very busy, these letters will mention the likelihood of a delay before we are able to contact them, and invite parents to contact us if they need to. This gives parents permission to call in for advice or to bring their child's name forward to be seen more quickly.

Case study

A parent called asking for her children to be seen urgently, as the funeral of their brother, who had been killed, was to take place the following week. The children did not know whether they wanted to view the body of their brother, and their deeply grieving parents were unable to have this conversation with them. The worker responded swiftly and met with the whole family for one session to explore the options. The children decided they wanted to view and say goodbye to their brother.

This way of working makes asks staff to:

- Make a working alliance very quickly
- Be flexible and accessible
- Work therapeutically within a short time frame

Once the referral has been allocated to a Candle worker, contact is made, and the first session is with the parent or carer, or occasionally with a social worker if the child is 'looked after'. This session functions both as another stage in the assessment, which has already begun with the phone contact and referral form, and a therapeutic meeting for the parent. The aim is to explore how the parent is, who is supporting them, what changes have happened in their lives, as well as how things have been for their children.

This session is often very long, as it may be the first time they have talked about their loss to a professional, and forges a bond between parent/carer and worker. We know from the research of the Harvard Child Bereavement Project (Worden 1996) and the work of Christ (2000) that the most significant factor for the child's bereavement process is the ability of the surviving parent or carer to function and support their child's grief, so the relationship with the parent is very important to us.

At the first meeting, parents are also given some information about Candle, and the way that we work is explained. Parents and children need frequent reminders that we only meet for six sessions, and staff tend to make appointments for three at a time, as many of our parents struggle to remember appointments. Sessions are offered at intervals that work best for the family, most are met weekly or fortnightly, but longer intervals are offered at times.

Children seem to be able to internalize the time scale more easily than parents, and are able to work well on their issues within a short time frame.

Some families attend for fewer than six sessions, as the work is completed in a shorter time. I have a check list in my mind that I use to evaluate the work I am doing with a child, based on the list of the needs of bereaved children which are for:

- Information about what has happened and what is likely to happen, delivered in a way that is truthful and simple
- Reassurance about their own anxieties
- A chance to name and express feelings
- Ways to hold onto memories
- Strategies to cope in a changed world
- Help for parents to help their children, now and in the future.
- Understanding that information will need to be repeated or revisited over time
- Being with adults who share their feelings
- Opportunities to reflect and remember with others.

(Monroe 1990)

How the sessions are structured is entirely the decision of the staff member and the family. Families come in all shapes and sizes, and the Candle team come from different training and experience backgrounds. What works best is what works for the particular combination of child and worker.

My own preferred style is to meet the family at reception and check out how things are with the parent as we walk through to the room, and then decide with them whether to meet the child alone first or to meet together, based on what has been happening for them since we last met. Following an individual session with a child, I meet with them and their parent informally, often over a coffee and give them general feedback about what we have been doing or discussing in the session. This general feedback does not breach the confidentiality agreement we have with the child as no details are given unless the child wishes us to, but I feel it is important that the parent or carer knows what has been the theme of the meeting. We aim to demystify and normalize the bereavement process and empower the parent with knowledge and information that will help their child. Working within a short time frame also requires a collaborative approach between parent and worker. The focus must always be on facilitating the parent to help their child, as the intervention is an introduction to a way of approaching and managing a process that will continue for a long time. Children grasp this idea very quickly, and are usually eager to tell their parent what has happened in the session, sometimes checking it out with me as they do so. I remind both parents and children about the number of sessions we have left, and always review the work we have done together in the final session with the child. In this way I hope to reinforce the learning for the child and give them a sense of achievement. I explain to them about the extended warranty, and give examples of when they might want to use it.

Case study

In the last session with a child of eight whose sister had died, we looked at the pictures she had drawn and talked through again the worries and fears she had about her parents. When I mentioned times she might feel she needed to return, she immediately responded;

'My sisters birthday is in the autumn term. I don't know what is going to happen'.

I was able to reassure her that she could come back if she needed to, and mentioned this to her parents when we all met together.

The final session also involves a ritualized ending, which is again done slightly differently by each Candle worker, but often involves a small gift to remind them of us, and a photograph taken with the worker for them to keep. The message to the child is of confidence in their ability to carry on with their life without us, using the things they have done in the sessions to support them, and knowing that they can come back if they need to.

How do families make contact again?

Parents and children are told together that if the child wants to make contact again they can ask their parent to contact us. This highlights the importance of a good working relationship with the parent, as they will need to be responsive to their child's needs and feel comfortable to call us. We work hard to make the project as accessible as possible, and encourage parents to make contact whenever they have a query connected to bereavement, reassuring them that all calls are welcome.

Another means of keeping contact are the ongoing parent/carer and young people's groups as described in Chapters 7 and 20. Parents and young people are known to the project, and sometimes request further intervention through the group leader, who takes it back to the staff team.

Bereaved families may need to make contact again with the project at times they can anticipate such as anniversaries or major changes such as moving house, as well when the unexpected arises. Later in the chapter an extended case study gives several examples of expected and unexpected instances when the warranty has been called on. One of the most frequent reasons for a renewed contact is school transition, which in the UK is when children are 10-11 years old. It is often a fraught time for families, as there are no guarantees of obtaining the first choice of secondary school. Many bereaved families find it particularly hard, as the children are leaving the safety of the known environment of the primary or elementary school, where they have often attended since starting school at four-five years old and where they will usually have one class teacher for most of the school day. Secondary schools are usually much larger, and children have lessons from many different subject teachers. Children often want to talk through how to manage the change.

Case study

Three children were left in the care of their grandparents after their mother was killed by their father. They were all seen in the project, and came back several times for a variety of reasons. As the criminal justice process unfolded they needed help with understanding the way it worked, and coping with the inevitable publicity. Their grandparents needed help with accessing their rights as carers for the children, and how to cope with contact with their father's family.

School transition was particularly important for the oldest child. They all attended the same small primary school, where they were well known and protected. He came to meet with me to discuss how to manage the transition. We talked about who he wanted to tell about his mother and how to do that, in the knowledge that there might be times that this would be important, as his father might ask the Court for leave to appeal his prison sentence.

Sometimes a letter from the project will assist a parent in a request for a school which will better support their bereaved child, whether because of its pastoral care reputation or for other reasons such as proximity to home. We are always happy to write if we feel it is appropriate.

Is the extended warranty transferable?

Candle has been in existence for 10 years to date (2008). The project has been fortunate in having a very stable staff team, which has grown slowly as demand and funding allowed. Staff members encourage families to make a relationship to the project and not only to the individual staff member, a process that is facilitated by the groupwork programme. Children and families attend groups where the worker they know may be not be part of the team leading the day, so have to make relationships with new Candle staff.

The system appears to work, as we receive referrals from families who know that the worker who met them originally has left, and readily accept intervention from another worker. This is usually myself, as I have been with the project longest and am likely to have some memory of the family through supervision. We have kept all the case notes since the project began, which provides background information, and an initial assessment phone call is made to find out what the current issues are.

Case study

A father and his five-year old son, who were bereaved by the suicide of his mother, were seen by a social work student on placement, who told them to contact me if they needed help in the future. Three years later, the father brought Ben into the reception and asked to see me. Ben, who was now eight had been crying a lot for no reason, and his father was very worried that he might be depressed. Ben's mother had had a diagnosis of manic depression, and had been very depressed when she took her own life. When we discussed this in more detail, Ben said that he had become very upset when his father had gone out recently to buy some milk and had taken a very long time. His father said that he had remembered more things he needed, and that he had tried to call Ben but had dialled the wrong number.

I reminded Ben and his father of how hard it must have been for Ben, who had memories still of going to bed one night and waking up to find his mother gone. He never saw her again. Ben's father was able to understand how very affected Ben was by this and how likely he was to find all separations difficult, and that he needed to reassure Ben very often. I explained to him that Ben was not likely to inherit his mother's manic depression, and that his tears were a normal way for a young child to express his worries about being separated from his much loved father.

Is the warranty always applicable?

Understandably, parents often call Candle when they have concerns about their children. The relationship is already established, and contact is made as easy as possible. The project receives a number of requests every year that are not really bereavement connected and we do our best to suggest more appropriate sources of help.

Some of the families we work with have many difficulties to cope with that pre-date the bereavement, and we have to be clear with referrers and with parents about the limits of our service. We are able to make a difference to the experience a child has of the bereavement process, but not able to address many other social, educational and practical issues that may have been a problem for some time.

Case study

A nine year old child who had been worked with two years previously when his grandmother had died was referred back to the project when he was about to be excluded from his school. His behaviour had been very difficult for a long time, and the bereavement had made it worse. Talking to his single parent mother, it became clear that his current behaviour problems did not relate to the loss of his grandmother but to her increasing difficulties in setting limits and establishing boundaries for a boy who was now physically and verbally quite threatening to her. The worker suggested alternative sources of support for her parenting.

A telephone assessment will often determine whether there is a bereavement issue, or if the difficulties need to be addressed by another agency, and we will give families names of agencies to contact. Even when we have to refuse further intervention from Candle, the opportunity to talk things through and signposting on to other agencies is a service that is appreciated. Agencies such as Child and Adolescent Mental Health services, voluntary agencies such as Youth Counselling Services, or local authority Children's Services appreciate a written report consisting of a brief introduction to the child, a clear account of the work that Candle has done, and a brief summary of our reasoning for referral on, and I believe that this constitutes a service for the child or family that we can and should offer.

Children are very capable of recognizing and using the extended warranty appropriately.

Case study

A young boy of eight asked his mother if he could see me again when the inquest into his father's death prompted extensive negative media coverage that included photographs of his father. Although his family had not bought the newspapers and did not watch the television news at the time, many others did, and he became very distressed at home and school. He needed to talk through his feelings and how to deal with them and to hear from his mother that she was intending to keep some of the newspaper articles for him to read with a close relative when he felt ready to.

Therapeutically, the question arises of how much to focus on the 'here and now' issues and how much on the 'there and then' of the bereavement. This is best illustrated by a description of work done with a family who drew on the extended warranty many times in the four years of their contact with Candle. In this example, I have asked special permission from this family to tell their story, and have only changed their names. In all other examples in the chapter I have used a number of methods to anonymize.

Case study

Barry's father Dave died in a collision on his motor bike in July 1999. He was on holiday with a friend, and the collision happened when he came off his bike on a bend in the road and was thrown onto an oncoming car. His neck was broken and he died instantly. His wife Carrie stayed up all night after hearing from the police, waiting to tell Barry the news.

Barry was five and a half and his sister Mary was two and a half when I first met the family in November 1999. Barry was a very bright and articulate child with a reading ability well above the normal range, and he was very close to his father. Barry was finding it hard to talk about his father and was having difficulties with temper tantrums that he found hard to control, which made him an easy target for teasing at school. His mother was also seeing a bereavement counsellor, which made it easier for Barry to accept his need for counselling. He used the six sessions well to talk about the good memories he had of his father, and Carrie felt that he had been able to open up more.

In March the following year, Barry attended a group day for children which he enjoyed very much although he was the youngest child present. In July, his mother referred him back to the project, as he had been very upset around the anniversary of the death. He had chosen to go to the school fete rather than attend a picnic with the other families from the Candle Project (see Chapter 7) and Carrie wondered if he had half expected to see his dad at the fete, as they had gone together the year before. Barry was very young when his father died, and it was quite possible that he did not fully understand the permanence of death. His immaturity was easy to miss, as he was so articulate and assured with adults. When we met he admitted that he had hoped to see his dad at the fete, and we discussed the scientific reasons that people cannot come back from the dead, touched on the resurrection of Jesus, and checked out with one of the St Christopher's doctors how the paramedics would have checked to see that Dave was actually dead. Barry then told me that he knew anyway that people could not come back as he was very clever. I have had some of the most difficult existential discussions of my professional career with bereaved children. They often demand to know my opinions and beliefs about issues I myself struggle with. I have always tried hard to be as honest as I can, although this has not always been the most comfortable answer for the child or for me.

Barry also told me in this meeting that he wanted mum to find another dad, that he would be nice to him whoever he was, as long as he looked like Barry. We discussed the uniqueness of his relationship with his dad, and when I spoke to Carrie she told me that her husband's best friend, Sam was now spending a lot of time with her and the children. Although she felt it was too early to think about a relationship, she could see that Barry was ahead of her.

The next contact came in November that year, when Barry asked to see me as he had become very upset as he realized that his father would not be there for Christmas. This had not really registered with him in the first year as things were still very recent, and the family were preoccupied with a planned trip to Australia, which happened just after Christmas. This year Barry was very angry that his dad would not be there to do all the things with him that the other children's fathers were doing. He drew a picture of a Christmas tree with decorations for everyone in the family including dad, and we talked about feelings for people who had died being very powerful at Christmas.

Barry, as with several of the children we worked with, was upset about the events of September 11th 2001. Children who experienced the sudden death of a parent or close relative were reminded and distressed by the TV footage of the sudden and traumatic deaths of so many other parents, and found themselves revisiting their own early reactions. Shortly after the attacks, his mother was due to attend a reception at the House of Commons with the Candle Project parents' group, and Barry was very anxious about her attending. Carrie talked to him about the extra security there would be in that particular building, and offered not to go if he was still worried. He thought it through and agreed to her attending.

In the spring of 2002, I saw Barry again as he wanted to talk about missing his dad, who was not there to tell him stories of what he had been was like when he was Barry's age. This is an example of the way in which a young child, (he was still only seven) gradually realizes the many different aspects of bereavement. I could only agree with him that it was hard to have to accept this, and say that I was sorry that it hurt. We discussed how he could ask Sam about dad, as he had been friends with him since childhood. Barry said that it was very nice to have Sam around, but not as good as dad.

In 2003 Carrie told me that she and Sam and the children had decided to move to Australia. The children were excited, but did not fully understand that the distances would mean saying goodbye to their friends. She had been attending the parents group since it began, and was sad to be leaving them as well. We arranged a final session in July to say goodbye.

The whole family came for what was a very emotional session. Barry told me that he felt leaving his home, which was very linked for him with his father, would be hardest for him and for Sam. He was the one most like his dad, and Sam had known his dad for so long. He told me again how he had been told the news of his father's death and cried, and how he had kept a bit of his motorbike, and that when he grew older he would buy the same sort of bike. He said the person he would miss most was one friend at school who reminded him a lot of his dad, and ended by telling me that his dad had been the best dad anyone could have had, and that 'the bond was going to be broken, but not too badly'. I was struck by his resourcefulness as he described ways he would hold on to memories, and his maturity as he talked about his link with his father.

Carrie had found the whole process leading up to the move very painful, as she was facing so many reminders. When her husband died she had not bothered to change the name on the TV licence, and when she called to cancel it was told that she would have to send in a copy of his death certificate. This year, for the first time, Barry had forgotten to make a card for fathers' day, and Mary had made one for Sam and asked him to be her dad. Carrie found this very difficult, as she herself was struggling with wanting to make a new life and move on but fearing that they would forget all that the old life had meant.

The family have now been in Australia for some years, and Carrie has emailed or telephoned me regularly to update me on their progress, and to ask for advice on expected and unexpected issues. The most recent contact was prompted by the news that she and Sam were intending to get married. She wanted to check through with me how to ask the children's permission, as both she and Sam felt that this was more important than the marriage.

Both children gave their permission and appreciated being consulted. Mary, although very happy with the news, spent some time writing letters to her father which she displayed in her bedroom, which Carrie thought were statements about her need to hold on to her memories and feelings for her birth father at a time of change. Barry has at times struggled with who and how to tell staff at school about his father. New staff understandably assume that the family they meet are all related, and children do not want to have to tell the story of a parent's death over and over again. Carrie spoke to him about how he was going to let his friends at school know about the marriage, and decided with him that she would speak to the school.

The contact I had with this family over a number of years demonstrates the importance of a service that is speedily accessible when needed. Children need space to consider strategies to cope with the changing demands of their lives as they grow and develop. The adults around them need opportunities to contact a service that has been helpful in the past if issues arise that they need help with. The service is rarely used inappropriately, and if it is the costs on staff time are small. Many families require only a telephone call. The knowledge that someone is available if necessary is in itself sufficient for some families, and allows them to make the decision about contact when they feel they really need it. Families appreciate the autonomy this gives them. The service Candle delivers is designed to promote the natural resilience in the families we see, by emphasizing their strengths and their capacity to overcome adversity. Over the time of a family's contact with us, that service will change in nature to respond to their changing circumstances. Given appropriate support and a good helping of luck, a family will come through bereavement strengthened by the experience and better able to cope with any other adversities that may arise.

References

Christ, G.H. (2000) *Healing Children's Grief*. Oxford: Oxford University Press.

Levy, J. (2004) Unseen support for bereaved families. *Bereavement Care*, **23**(2): 25–26.

Monroe, B. (1990) Supporting children facing bereavement. In Saunders, C. (ed). *Hospice and Palliative Care: An Interdisciplinary Approach*. London: Edward Arnold. pp78–84.

Monroe, B. (1997) *The Development of a Hospice Consultancy Service* (abstract). EAPC Conference. London.

Stokes, J.A. (2004) *Then Now and Always*. Cheltenham: Winston's Wish.

Worden, J.W. (1996) *Children and Grief: When a Parent Dies*. New York: The Guilford Press.

Chapter 12

Schools and grief: attending
to people and place[1]

Louise Rowling

Introduction

Focusing on schools as physical and psychosocial places addresses the current imbalance in our understanding of loss and grief interventions that can support children and young people. The interventions that are needed are not just individual and personal but include a significant social context of their lives – the school community. An extensive review of the literature on young people's bereavement identified the acknowledgement of their social worlds as a gap in existing research and practice (Ribbens McCarthy 2006). This chapter aims to address this deficiency by drawing on various theoretical perspectives, empirical research, and practical examples to elucidate the school community's role in supporting its bereaved school community members.

In the past schools have been characterized by bereavement service professionals chiefly as functional places for interventions, for example describing their interventions as 'working in schools'. Yet an extensive body of interdisciplinary work theorizing 'sense of place' delineates important qualities of places (such as schools) as being seen more than sites or geographic spaces for interventions. The theory of place and its empirical work provides direction for a school community focus. Drawing on the work of Proshansky (1978) a school community's place identity can be identified as reflecting an individual's unique experience and socialization, as well as those experiences common to all individual and school group members. Applying a public health approach provides an additional lens for a more holistic 'individual within their psychosocial environment' orientation (International Working Group on Death, Dying and Bereavement).

Further support for a broader focus for interventions comes from shifts in the loss and grief field particularly in relation to children and adolescents.

---

[1] Many of the ideas in this chapter are delineated in greater detail in Rowling, L (2003) *Grief in school communities: effective support strategies*, Buckingham, Open University Press.

Over the past decade or so, global terrorism and violence have become part of the everyday lives of individuals, communities, and nation states, not only because of the exposure given to events by the global media coverage, but also due to the targeting of previously 'safe' environments such as: workplaces, social gatherings in clubs and hotels, and schools. A critical point in terms of potential impact on people in this exposure is the intimacy in the reporting of these tragic events. It is these events and their reporting that has contributed to experiences of loss, either real or vicarious, becoming as in times past, a more mainstream part of life in Western communities. That is, these events and experiences are ceasing to be seen as private individual or family matters. In this wider societal context the need for dual processes of community recovery and individual and family support becomes imperative.

Reconceptualizing grief as a globalized as well as local personal phenomenon provides the opportunity to move it from an individualised pathologized experience, the purview of the counselling profession, to a 'normal' life event where restorative community processes provide support (Rowling 2003). Viewed from this perspective loss can be placed not only in a psychological framework with concomitant individual and group support processes, but within the aegis of public health and social institutions such as faith communities and schools. This wider framing facilitates understanding the impact these events can have on school community members when the sense of safety, trust, and predictability of life for people in the environments of their everyday worlds is disrupted.

Approaches from public health – interdisciplinary, holistic and capacity building, and the health promoting school (healthy schools) underpin this chapter. A public health approach focuses on the school community that acknowledges linkages between people and place and how organizational conditions can be created that enhance the positive outcomes of connectedness to school as a place for individuals and groups.

Validating, restorative and enfranchising approaches need to be created in school communities. A reorientation of practices of service providers may be needed in short term interventions within this framework.

Individuals in the context of their school community

Individuals and groups have been the focus of much of the research and interventions in the field of thanatology. The immediate needs individuals present are undoubtedly a powerful basis for theorizing, research and for developing effective interventions. But for children and young people, by concentrating on an individual's experience divorced from its context, we have failed to embed their issues of concern in a social environment. For most young people, after the family, this environment involves the school community. Additionally there has often been too much of a focus on the pathology of grief. It could be argued that this focus has been necessary to establish grief as a legitimate area through comprehensive research and practice. But it is time to re-conceptualize the area, from a concentration on individuals' experiences to an equal place in the research and practice for the contextual variables within which the bereavement occurs. This chapter examines the role of the school as a social place and a community institution. In this environment young people can look to schools as places to:

- help define the reality of their losses;
- express feelings associated with them;
- help create meaning of their loss;
- provide support and access to information; and
- help integrate the experience into their lives (Rowling 2003).

The school is not only a social institution for young people; it is also a workplace for staff, all of whom spend many hours there. It can provide an environment (in terms of policies, programmes and practices) that is experienced as supportive as well as access to individuals who can provide help through formal and informal mechanisms.

The contribution of the theory of place to enhancing understanding of psychosocial context (Galliano and Loeffler 1999; Proshansky 1978, 1983; Turner and Turner 2006) lies in its delineation of elements that help expand our understanding of a holistic view of the students and their school environments. One element of place theory is 'place identity'. This involves an individual or a group's 'environmental past' (Proshansky 1983) which includes images and memories of places, conscious and unconscious beliefs, expectations, feelings, preferences and interactions in and with physical settings. That is, any given interaction a student, teacher, or principal may have in the physical setting is created within a collection of expectations, beliefs, feelings, ideas and aspirations about that setting. In this way the meaning function of the setting – what should happen in it, what the setting is supposed to be like, and how the individual and others are supposed to behave in it, is assigned.

Another element of place theory is sense of place. This has been described by Galliano and Loeffler (1999) as comprising of personal memory, community history, physical and landscape appearance, and emotional attachment. More recently Turner and Turner (2006) have delineated the components of a sense of place as:

- physical characteristics of the environment;
- affect and meanings including memories and associations;

♦ activities of people in the place; and

♦ social interactions associated with the place (p207).

These components expand the elements identified by Ribbens McCarthy (2006) that provide the hinge between public and private faces of bereavement. In particular they point to the dynamic interactions of the person in their physical and social context and the potential impact of the memories and associations of that interaction on the meanings of bereavement experiences. The importance of this expanded understanding of schools as significant places in the lives of school community members is that bereavement interventions need to be cognisant of all the 'place' components that could be affected by and influence new meanings, emotional responses, behaviours, social interactions, and school history. This is especially important if the loss involves intrusion of the school physical and psychosocial space.

A validating community

The emphasis in this chapter is on building the capacity of the school community to achieve a comprehensive approach to the grief experiences of its members. This wider whole school system of care is a preventive approach that involves the school organization, ethos and environment, partnerships and services and curriculum (Fig. 12.1). The loss experiences of teachers and students can be validated through provision of pastoral care processes, curriculum, critical incident management plans, and policies; and special leave policies for staff. Silverman and Worden (1992) identified that following the death of a parent, children who received support at home and in school displayed fewer behavioural problems than those who did not have similar support networks.

Current global evidence in school health and well-being no longer concentrates on the curriculum as the sole focus for bringing about health behaviour change in schools. The comprehensive approach to school health and well-being embodied in the health promoting schools framework or healthy schools, acknowledges the wider impact of the psychosocial environment in the school as well as the contribution of family and community. Addressing loss and grief in schools by action in each of the health promoting school areas creates a supportive context.

Health promoting schools is also more than addressing health issues in schools in a comprehensive way – such as creating policy to support curriculum or changing the physical environment. It involves providing the conditions for the empowerment of the school community to take ownership of the health of its community, thereby being proactive for health issues, rather than being reactive to events as they occur. This approach has significant implications for outside service providers. They may need to shift their work practices from a sole focus

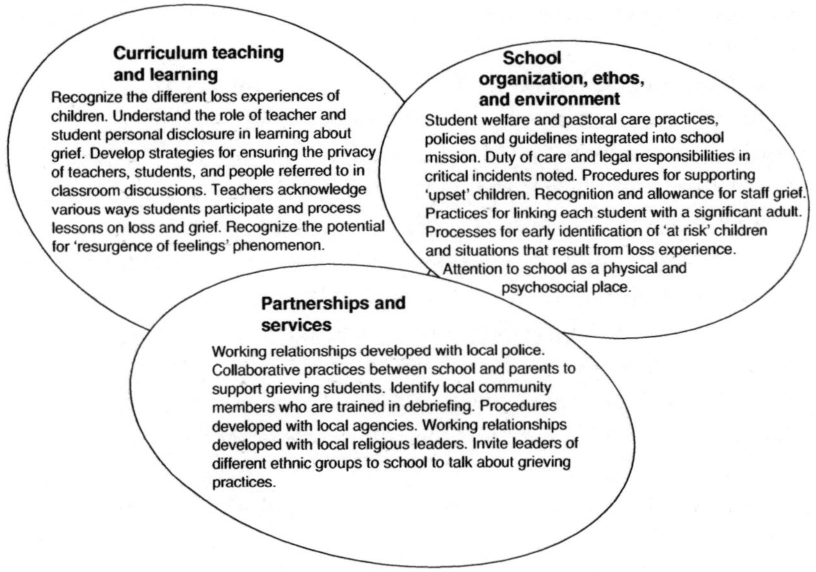

Curriculum teaching and learning

Recognize the different loss experiences of children. Understand the role of teacher and student personal disclosure in learning about grief. Develop strategies for ensuring the privacy of teachers, students, and people referred to in classroom discussions. Teachers acknowledge various ways students participate and process lessons on loss and grief. Recognize the potential for 'resurgence of feelings' phenomenon.

School organization, ethos, and environment

Student welfare and pastoral care practices, policies and guidelines integrated into school mission. Duty of care and legal responsibilities in critical incidents noted. Procedures for supporting 'upset' children. Recognition and allowance for staff grief. Practices for linking each student with a significant adult. Processes for early identification of 'at risk' children and situations that result from loss experience. Attention to school as a physical and psychosocial place.

Partnerships and services

Working relationships developed with local police. Collaborative practices between school and parents to support grieving students. Identify local community members who are trained in debriefing. Procedures developed with local agencies. Working relationships developed with local religious leaders. Invite leaders of different ethnic groups to school to talk about grieving practices.

Fig. 12.1 Loss and grief in the health promoting school framework (Rowling 2003).

on crisis intervention to include working to create proactive partnerships with school communities. These partnerships need to involve actively working with school personnel to tailor support to meet their expressed needs and changing roles from grief experts to facilitators and supporters of school actions.

Conceptualizing loss and grief within the social environment of the school is a theoretically and practically sound strategy. It acknowledges the role of the school organizational factors that can facilitate the creation of a context that accepts the 'normality of grief'. This is in contrast to a crisis orientated approach which may fail to recognize the school as a community, a social place, which has the capacity to provide support (Petersen and Straub 1992). Within this place there can be behaviours and interactions that sanction or block young people's experience of grief.

School organization, ethos, and environment

A holistic approach to loss and grief involves the hidden curriculum or the ethos of the school. Identifying this is not easy. The ethos of a supportive context includes: the school policies that provide for the emotional well-being of students; a well developed pastoral care system; clear procedures for referral of students to outside agencies; availability of a school-based counselling service; and/or a grief support programme. The ethos also involves staff relationships – how the school cares for its staff; recognition of the importance of maintaining staff morale; and the relationships between the Head Teacher and individual staff members.

Validation of grief can occur through the purposeful practices offering different types of support – emotional, informational, practical and social (Rowling 2003). Emotional support arises from actions focused on individuals such as the acknowledgement of feelings of sadness so that children are allowed time out from lessons and/or providing opportunities to express those feelings in art, writing, or through vigorous physical activity. Social support comes from the sense of communal caring and connectedness in shared rituals, or from school structures such as special grief support groups conducted in the school. Instrumental and practical support for a bereaved teacher could come from colleagues who take his or her classes and extra duties, or from school practices that allow staff to take an informal leave during periods of grief.

Being part of the 'hidden curriculum', the school ethos and the attendant belief system that is the basis of a supportive environment may need to be made explicit. Statements from school leaders that represent the underlying beliefs and philosophies of school practices and policies are one way of achieving this explicitness.

Sensitive issues such as loss and grief create debate and disagreement in school communities. This is due to their characteristics of emotionality, values, beliefs, and past experience combined with the varying perspectives of school community members (Rowling 1996 2003). Some researchers report that substantial proportions of young people do not want schools involved in such personal and private issues (Ribbens McCarthy 2006). However this finding is not universal. There are cultural differences in preparedness to discuss and seek support (Rowling and Holland 2000). As well as the differences in research outcomes that can partially be explained by research methodology problems (viz lack of delineation of time frames for self report after a significant loss; adults reporting on childhood experiences; and lack of differentiation in male/female responses). Yet young people learning about loss and grief offer a more considered response. In replying to a question about the group learning about loss and grief (where the researcher was a participant observer in the session) these 16 year olds stated[2]:

> You have to talk about it, be aware of it. It is not something you can take easily.
> It gives you ideas about how to explain yourself if you were in that situation, to watch what they are doing.

---

[2] Verbatim anonymised responses are from research more fully reported in Rowling (2003).

I was surprised that we did talk about death but it was a good topic, although it isn't a nice thought though.

I was pleased we talked about a variety of topics especially death as it helped me understand about death and how we can cope with our grief and others grief.

(Rowling 2003)

A school's concern about students' personal well-being will be evident in implementation of policies for handling sensitive issues. For example, a critical incident management plan (Yule and Gold 1993) demonstrates a school's commitment to the well-being of school community members if a traumatic incident occurs. It is a demonstration of a school's caring ethos. Similarly inclusive practices can acknowledge varying mourning rituals of different faith communities. Or clear guidelines can be in operation to handle confidentiality and privacy issues for young people. Less obvious policies include assessment policies, where the impact of grief for adolescents that may affect their school performance should be noted. This impact may be immediate, but it can also be delayed, affecting schoolwork months after the loss.

Partnerships and services

The second area of the health promoting school framework concerns the development of partnerships. These partnerships are with parents as well as outside agencies. Well developed partnerships with outside agencies provide the school with ready access to personnel for referral of 'at risk' students or staff traumatized by violence or other critical incidents. These relationships also provide resources that can assist in educating families, who can then be more supportive and understanding of the experience of their grieving children and siblings. Similarly partnerships with ethnic and religious leaders bring opportunities for the school to work with these community leaders for support of families.

Small groups with trained facilitators from bereavement support services can provide short term interventions either on the school grounds and in school time or outside school hours. These support programmes can be helpful for children (Smith and Pennells 1995). But there is also a real need for dialogue with young people – what do they see as helpful? How do they experience events? Dialogue also needs to be encouraged about young people, between service providers and school personnel. Whilst some school personnel and service providers may worry this would jeopardise confidentiality, protocols that elaborate confidentiality versus privacy can help overcome this fear. In this way young people who participate in short term interventions can be supported in the longer term by school personnel as they adjust to their loss.

The technical expertise of bereavement agencies needs to be employed to support school communities in their efforts to address loss and grief. Unless this happens, children's grief will continue to be handled ineffectively. It will still be seen as 'abnormal' and therefore solely the role of psychologists or social workers.

Curriculum

In a caring community that validates grief experiences, a very real concern for teachers is – how to respond to an upset child. Setting up procedures to manage such occurrences needs to be done as part of the whole school approach and especially before lessons are taught (Rowling 2003).

Different classroom teaching approaches to loss and grief education are being adopted. In Australia teaching is occurring in a larger mental health promotion framework. It is proactive in that it is not developed after a crisis but included as a part of existing mental health programmes built around common skill areas such as help seeking, and addressing stigma to enable individuals to cope, seek help and/or to be supportive to others (Rowling 2003). This is a natural way to incorporate exploration of feelings of grief and experiences associated with loss. This approach facilitates the normalization of grief through education (Zisook 1987). Mental preparation and planning, before a death or other critical event occurs, leads to a much better handling than if one 'takes things as they come'.

In England death and loss have been programmed in the National Curriculum in PSHE/citizenship (Ribbens McCarthy 2006). The National Children's Bureau (Job and Frances 2004) have provided extensive curriculum and pastoral care advice. There is also specific support from the Department of Health for the inclusion of death and bereavement in the curriculum. How far these recommendations have been implemented has not been determined (Ribbens McCarthy 2006).

Training for teachers to teach about loss and grief, and the active learning styles utilized, is necessary. The sensitivity in the teaching is a result of the personal experiences of teachers, the pedagogy, and the content. There are professional challenges for teachers in responding to students who get upset when they disclose emotional life events that are triggered by the lesson. In these instances a teacher needs to develop expertise in balancing the aims of the lessons with creating an open and trusting environment where students feel comfortable to share their experiences. Keeping this balance is a formidable task for teachers especially when approaching these lessons for the first time (Rowling 2003).

Students respond positively to teachers who are prepared to devote time to issues that impact on their lives, issues that families and some communities can treat as taboo topics. The result of these taboos is that many young people still grieve silently and alone. School education is needed to increase acceptance by a young person's peers of the impact of loss. To achieve this children and adolescents need to be taught about loss and grief as a normal part of their education, so that they can understand their own experiences and limit the sanctions that they apply to their peers.

Allan reported that he felt his friends understood his situation. His mother was very ill. She had frequent life threatening fits that often required immediate treatment. He needed to be at home in the evening in case his mother needed help. He had accepted this and so had his friends:

> Most of my friends understand. They ask me to sleep over and I say 'No'. They know I have a good reason for staying home and looking after Mum.

> (Allan, 14 years old)

Teachers may feel ill-equipped to manage loss issues and view this role as one more thing they are being asked to do. They may see themselves as a teacher of a subject and in comparison to bereavement service providers, that they lack expert knowledge that they perceive as needed to manage grief issues. Despite this they are concerned about issues that impact on children's academic achievement. A child's school work is likely to be affected by bereavement (Corr and Balk 1999), so loss and grief has academic outcomes as well as emotional and social.

Service providers have a significant role to play in providing technical support to teachers and modelling effective teaching pedagogy. This may involve being open to hearing young people's experiences, providing answers to questions frequently asked (viz what happens when you die?), and team teaching to increase a teacher's confidence and comfort level. A support team to staff teaching in the area is necessary to defuse issues that might arise for the teacher, for example a teacher feeling guilty if students become distressed in the classroom as a result of the lesson.

Training is necessary for teachers to develop skills and knowledge about loss and grief as well as how to teach effectively in this area (Rowling 2003). With this training, teachers can be supportive to families particularly to those who are isolated in the community. In this way a sense of place, belonging and connection to the school community can be created. This can facilitate natural recovery processes for the family.

Despite the personal and professional challenges teachers do acknowledge grief in their students' lives, and believe that teaching all students about grief as a life experience is part of their role as a teacher. They see it as relating to students so that they feel confident in the learning situation, a necessary state if they are to achieve their educational goals (Rowling 2003).

A restorative community

As well as the preventive approach of a whole school system of care, there may be need for additional action for a longer term restoration of the school if violence has invaded not only individuals' lives, but also affecting the geographic space and the social environment of the school.

Violation of school can involve destruction of a sense of safety. Feelings of safety therefore need to be recreated, the school being reclaimed as an environment where order, structure and predictability facilitate the daily routines of teaching and learning. Reclaiming rituals allow for feelings to be collectively constructed and expressed through actions. They create a space, a structure with boundaries where school community members can feel safe to express their tears or reflect on their inner sadness. It is also a place where a sense of hope and faith in the future can be initiated. School leaders can provide guidance for the community response especially where there is confusion, anger and doubt. For example Matt, a head teacher, described the feeling he had when he walked into his school grounds after a young man unconnected to the school had hanged himself in the playground:

> They [the school community] felt very, very intruded upon. And the gravity of having someone commit suicide where you spend a lot of your time pumping emotional energy into, it is very, very difficult. Adults had to reclaim the place for the kids and that was my role to start the process of reclaiming the place for the school community.

> (Matt, head teacher 17 years)

Similarly in another school, a student was murdered on the way home from school along a familiar shortcut frequented by many students. The students, with the help of the local government public works department and the wider community, cleared the track of vegetation and lighting was installed. A formal pathway was declared for the school and the students organized a dedication ceremony. It was through this collective action that the students expressed their grief and reclaimed the violated space. Teachers who bring parents and families into these restorative activities, allowing contact and engagement with their child's peers, can facilitate the recovery process for the family. The memories of connectedness and safety generated by rituals created by students and other school community members can provide reassurance long after the ceremonies have occurred. Young people need social practices available to them to make their grief visible. Yet few are available to them (Ribbens McCarthy 2006). School-organized rituals can help fulfil this need.

An enfranchising community

The outcome for staff and students where their school community is not validating and restorative is that they can be disenfranchised grievers. Disenfranchised grief is defined as: 'the grief that persons experience when they incur a loss that is not or cannot be openly acknowledged, publicly mourned, or socially supported. (Doka 1989 p4)

There are five triggers for disenfranchised grief:

The relationship is not recognized;

The loss is not recognized;

Society does not give the person that role; (Doka 1989)

The circumstances of the loss;

The ways individuals grieve (Doka 2002).

There are a number of sources of disenfranchised grief in a school community – self, others, and the social world of the school. Whilst there are similarities between schools, each school is unique with its own history, relationships, rules and procedures that often reflect particular cultural and religious values, beliefs. and normative behaviour. This is especially important because meanings about loss experiences (cognitive representations of reality) come from the culture and others' expectations mediated through an individual's internal resources and life experience and the school environment (Rowling 2002).

For young people there are different ways their grief is disenfranchised. These can be intrapersonal, interpersonal and environmental. Intrapersonal sources include fear of social disapproval; fear of loss of control linked to their emerging independence; and the current beliefs, perceptions and interpretations of their world. Young males in particular are subject to disenfranchisement due to the varying ways they process grief (Martin and Doka 2000). For them psycho-education, information giving about the normality of grief; classroom discussions about loss and grief; and the 'hearing of others' stories' provides a structure for their thinking, a way to process their grief. It is important to recognize that young men may not talk about their experiences and feelings, but they can still be processing and organizing their thoughts, as Ricardo (17 years old) described:

> It is good to hear about what others are saying. You can just sit there and listen and you have a conversation with yourself, in your mind, you turn it over and that helps. It gives you ideas about how you might explain yourself if you were in that situation.

> (Rowling 2002)

What is needed are school environments that validate the varying ways of expressing grief, sanctioning options for young males of diversion and reflection

(Martin and Doka 2000) processing by action rather than verbally expressing feeling; by thinking it through rather than talking.

For young people, two sources of interpersonal disenfranchisement are parents and peers. Peer relationships exemplify the paradox of disenfranchised grief. Peers can provide support by words and action but these mechanisms also do the disenfranchising. To address this education needs to occur with peers concurrently with provision of support to the griever.

The third source of disenfranchisement is their environment, the organizational rules about grieving and the wider school community practices about responding to losses. The extra threat posed by society's attitudes to young people, who are already vulnerable because of a loss experience and developmental challenges, creates a triple burden (Rowling 2002). Additionally adults may believe it is not the school's role to be proactive in creating a school place, where grief is normal and grieving acceptable (Rowling 1999; Rowling and Holland 2000).

Mental health professionals, bereavement counsellors, and educational psychologists in supporting young people experiencing disenfranchised grief need to ask 'What does the griever need to do? What changes are needed in the social environment, from adults, peers, family members, helping professionals and the wider community?' There needs to be recognition of the different pathways that young people follow as they learn to cope. Consequently different interventions will be required for different styles of grieving and different circumstances. Working with individuals will not address the behaviour of their peers towards their loss nor the organizational practices that disenfranchise school community members (Rowling 2002).

Research conducted about 15 years ago identified teachers as disenfranchised grievers (Rowling 1995). This influences their capacity to be supportive. Teaching is a profession where emotional connections are made: it is based on human interactions. Teachers care for their pupils. There exists the belief amongst teachers that you have to hide your emotions to manage a class, when a death occurs (Rowling 1995). For teachers there is a real fear of 'breaking down in front of the class'. If something traumatic occurs it is likely to involve intense emotions, often emotions that teachers themselves may not recognize. Being affected by grief and therefore not being able to perform their teaching role, influences a teacher's view of themselves as competent professionals because of the need to feel in control of the situation and to rise above natural emotional responses. From an organizational perspective, it is essential to create a supportive workplace for all school personnel.

In the management of an incident in a school, there needs to be recognition of the history of the school, particularly where events have occurred with their potential to revive memories. Support, the social sanctioning of grief, needs to be embedded in the school's normal processes.

Conclusion

In conclusion, adopting a comprehensive approach means we accept grief as a life event and as a legitimate area of concern for schools. Rather than seeing loss and grief as a special 'one off' experience it is mainstreamed into educational policy, and practice, and employment standards, as well as established as a wider health issue.

From an educational perspective a comprehensive strategy establishes proactive approaches which assist in:

- creating physical and psychosocial safety;
- demonstrating a school community's caring and responsible behaviour and thereby minimizing litigation threats; and
- helping ensure the public perception of schools as safe, physical and psychosocial places.

It is only coordination and cooperation that can create a healing community needed for young people.

There is enough research evidence and collective wisdom from professionals and young people to warrant comprehensive action by school communities. However there still needs to be care taken 'to do no harm' and to utilize the technical expertise of bereavement agencies combined with the insight, understanding and judgement of school personnel. Importantly the voices of young people need to be sought, included and valued. If school communities respond appropriately to loss, crises, and trauma that affect the young, learning becomes social and emotional as well as academic.

References

Becker, C., Clark, E., DeSpelder, L.A. et al. (In Review). A call to action: An IWG Charter for a Public Health Approach to Dying, death and loss.

Corr, C. and Balk, D. (eds) (1996) *Handbook of Adolescent Death and Bereavement.* New York: Springer.

Doka, K. (1989) (ed) *Disenfranchised Grief: Recognising Hidden Sorrow.* Lexington, Massachusetts: Lexington Books.

Doka, K. (2002) *Disenfranchised Grief: New Directions, Challenges and Strategies for Practice.* Champaign Ill: Research Press.

Galliano, S.J. and Loeffler, G.M. (1999) *Place Assessment: How People Define. Ecosystems.* General Technical Report. PNW-GTR-462. Portland, OR: U.S. Department of Agriculture, Forest Service, Pacific Northwest Research Station.

International Working Group on Death Dying and bereavement http://www.iwgddb.org/ (accessed 29th July, 2009).

Job, N. and Frances, G. (2004) *Childhood Bereavement: Developing the Curriculum and Pastoral Support.* London: National Children's Bureau.

Martin, T.I. and Doka, K.J. (2000) *Men Don't Cry ... Women do: Transcending Gender Stereotypes of Grief.* Philadelphia: Bruner Mazel.

Petersen, S. and Straub, R.L. (1992) *School Crisis Survival Guide: Management Techniques and Materials for Counsellors and Administrators.* West Nyack, New York: Centre for Applied Research in Education.

Proshansky, H.M. (1976) Environmental psychology and the real world. *American Psychologist,* **31**: 303–310.

Proshansky, H.M., Fabian, A.K., and Kaminoff, R. (1983) Place-identity: physical world socialization of the self. *Journal of Environmental Psychology,* **3**: 57–83.

Ribbens McCarthy, J. (2006) *Young People's Experiences of Loss and Bereavement.* England: Open University Press.

Rowling, L. (1995) Disenfranchised grief of teachers, *Omega. Journal of Death and Dying,* **31**: 317–329.

Rowling, L. (1996) A comprehensive approach to handling sensitive issues in schools with special reference to loss and grief. *Pastoral Care in Education,* **4**: 17–21.

Rowling, L. (1999) The role of policy in creating a supportive social context for the management of loss experiences and critical incidents in school communities. *Crisis, Illness and Loss,* **7**: 252–265.

Rowling, L. and Holland, J. (2000) Grief and school communities: the impact of social context, a comparison between Australia and England. *Death Studies,* 24: 35–50.

Rowling, L. (2002) Youth and disenfranchised grief. In Doka, K. (ed) *Disenfranchised Grief: New Directions, Challenges and Strategies for Practice.* Champaign Ill: Research Press.

Rowling, L. (2003) *Grief in School Communities: Effective Support Strategies.* Buckingham: Open University Press.

Silverman, P.R. and Worden, J.W. (1992) Children's reactions to the death of a parent in the early months after the death. *American Journal of Orthopsychiatry,* **62**: 93–104.

Smith, S. and Pennells, M. (1995) *Interventions with Bereaved Children.* London: Jessica Kingsley Publications.

Turner, P. and Turner, S. (2006) Place, sense of place and presence. *Presence,* **15**(2): 204–217.

Yule, W. and Gold, A. (1993) *Wise Before the Event: Coping with Crises in School.* London: Calouste Gulbenkian Foundation.

Zisook, S. (ed) (1987) *Biopsychosocial Aspects of Bereavement.* United States of America: American Psychiatric Press.

Chapter 13

Seasons for Growth: a grief education programme helping children and young people deal with loss and change

Kate Macleod*

What does the Seasons for Growth Programme do?

- Aims to support young people to understand and manage the grief that is experienced because of the loss of a parent or significant other through death, separation, or divorce
- Assists in normalizing the emotions associated with loss
- Encourages the expression of thoughts and emotions
- Educates about the grief process
- Develops a peer support network
- Helps restore self-confidence and self esteem
- Draws on extensive research in developing a sound educative response to loss and grief.

Seasons for Growth emerged after an extensive research and consultation period by Good Grief Australia in1994-95. This identified a significant gap in support for children suffering loss and change and that there was a strong requirement for an educationally based programme which could be delivered safely, creatively, with cultural sensitivity and was underpinned by sound theory. The programme aims to produce a sense of resilience, personal growth, and acceptance of change in people's lives using William Worden's task- centred theory of the grieving process (Worden 1996). The programme is well-established in Australia, New Zealand, and Scotland.

* With acknowledgement to Moira Sugden for her support.

Programme structure: Companion training

The role of the Companion is fundamental to the Seasons process. Essentially Companions are committed individuals who can relate well to young people, listen effectively, have the ability to deal with their own feelings about loss and, importantly, have a sense of humour. Companions accompany the children and young people through the group process and themselves represent examples of people who have coped with change and loss in their own lives. Line management endorsement is expected in anticipation of agency support to allow the trained Companion time and resources to implement the programme and to ensure all trainees have been through Child Protection clearance.

A two-day training course, facilitated by Seasons Trainers, introduces the Companions to Worden's theory and its link to the Seasons model. In providing and modelling a safe environment, through self reflection and discussion, trainee Companions focus on recognizing reactions to loss and promoting coping strategies. Schools are often anxious to support pupils who have experienced loss but staff may not feel they have the skills. Seasons for Growth training provides a safe framework for those working with children to explore with sensitivity this emotionally challenging area of work. Companions come from a range of professional backgrounds including teachers, home-link workers, pupil support, social workers, school nurses, and committed volunteers.

The seasons framework using Worden's model

Worden's theoretical approach identifies four tasks which the programme links to the four seasons; 1) to accept the reality of loss – autumn; 2) to work through the pain of grief – winter; 3) to adjust to an environment in which the significant person is no longer present – spring; and 4) emotionally relocate the person and move on with life – summer. Within this framework children and young people are supported by trained Companions to share loss experiences, focusing on change as a natural part of life and promoting their awareness of coping strategies.

For example, the linking of Autumn with Worden's task of accepting the reality of loss acknowledges that there are times of disbelief and denial. Likening this to the highs (Halloween, and bonfires, and changing autumn colours), and lows of the season (but leaves die and days get shorter and darker, there is a chill in the air, misty mornings and stormy weather present ever changing challenges) helps the children to begin to recognize that change has a cycle. Adjustments need to be made in response to change both in our lives and in anticipation of Winter and darker times ahead.

With the second task of experiencing the pain of loss, the physical sensations of grieving are likened to how we find coping mechanisms in Winter to deal with the cold numbing times, when we may be more isolated from supports and comfort. Spring brings many changes of a more positive kind, but late frosts remind us that Winter is still not far away. Positive choices can be made about how to cope with difficult times and, crucially, learning from one another helps to lessen isolation. Summer is usually a time of feeling more relaxed and reflective, as with Worden's fourth task, which encourages memory work and continuing bonds (Klass 1999).

Worden's model encourages us to acknowledge that the process of grieving may not be a linear and staged experience. Seasons change and come around again, bereavement confronts us with many feelings and experiences that come and go, but we can learn the skills needed to cope with difficult emotions. The more you are aware of a task needing to be done, the better you get at it. The task -centred approach, focusing on dealing with feelings and reactions, acknowledges that everyday experiences will bring different feelings to the surface. It helps to explain behaviour as a consequence of difficult feelings, which lie under the surface but need to be 'claimed, named, tamed, and aimed' (as the programme suggests) towards more adaptive ways of coping. Recognizing that certain events, anniversaries, and family occasions will trigger emotional and behavioural responses, children can learn from one another that these reactions are normal. With time and anticipation of how events affect them, the young people can with growing confidence find acceptable and positive ways of coping.

Through a wide range of creative learning activities, the Seasons for Growth programme develops life skills in communication, decision- making, and problem solving while simultaneously encouraging peer communication and support. It assists young people to understand that their reactions to loss are normal. Companions have found it a positive experience to support bereaved children along with those who have other significant changes through separation and divorce. The losses may be different but the feelings tend to be the same.

Although Worden's model provides the focus and link to the Seasons, experienced professionals will find resonance with other supportive approaches, for example continuing bonds (Klass 1999) and the dual process model (Stroebe and Schut 1999). It is important to stress that Seasons for Growth does not provide individual therapy or counselling although evaluations point to the experience as being therapeutic to the group members.

How the programme works

The programme consists of five levels (ages 6-18 years), with three levels aimed at primary school pupils and two at secondary pupils. Companions have manuals, which guide them with a step-by-step plan for each session. Well designed personal journals with age appropriate exercises allow the children and young people to work through the Seasons, tackling issues relating to their loss experience, telling their own story, identifying how loss has affected them physically, emotionally and spiritually, and then sharing ways of coping. Confidentiality in the group setting is stressed, and the sharing of experiences through peer support helps the young people reflect that, on hearing others' stories, they are not alone.

The model has developed with two Companions working together facilitating the young people through eight sessions. There are two sessions per Season, lasting about an hour each. There is also a Celebration at the end of the programme, when young people can invite their parents/carers and a friend along to learn about the work they have done together. Craft work, art, mime, storytelling, and writing all feature in the programme and memory work allows the young people to appreciate the value of balanced memorializing of the person who is no longer physically present. A constant feature of the programme is to present the 'I can' philosophy, not letting the 'if onlys' dominate life and hinder adaptation to changing circumstances.

Ideally children and young people dealing with loss and change are best helped in their own communities, thus promoting avenues of support and an ongoing sense of connectedness. Throughout Scotland there are a range of ways Seasons is being promoted in communities, primarily with schools endorsing the programme thus allowing the young people to be supported by Companions known to them at school (Fig. 13.1). The model is also used by Companions in hospice settings and by voluntary agencies (Brown 2007) supporting vulnerable children. Parents and carers are given information on the programme and process, and the young people are then invited to consider joining a Seasons group. In schools and communities where Seasons is well-embedded, young people are now self referring as they hear of the positive experiences of their peers.

Does the programme work?

The Australian programme has been independently evaluated a number of times by respected Australian academics (Good Grief Australia). The evaluations concluded with the following outcomes:

- Seasons for Growth has a strong and positive effect on young people
- Parents, Companions, school principals, and agency managers believe without exception that the programme is beneficial to participants
- Young people said the programme had removed their sense of isolation, allowed them to express their feelings without being ashamed, and helped them to develop trust in others

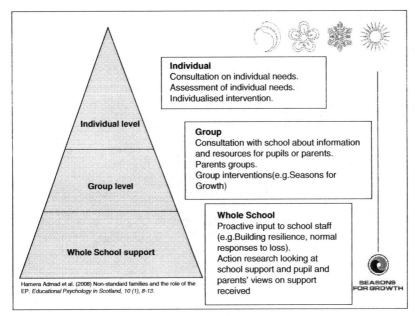

Fig. 13.1 Where does it fit in?

- Seasons for Growth contributes broadly to intervention against youth suicide (also supported by Choose Life, Scotland's National Suicide Prevention Policy) in that it provides an early system of safety, opportunities for identification and referral, thus lessening vulnerability

- Monitoring and evaluation are strong elements of the whole programme. Companions monitor and evaluate their planning and performance throughout the sessions, and the young people and their parents/carers are all invited to evaluate the effectiveness of the programme.

In Scotland the Notre Dame Centre collates evaluations to ensure the ongoing validity of the experience for children and young people, and these reflect the outcomes of the Australian evaluation.

Examples of exercises promoting positive outcomes

An important element of the first session is to make the link to the seasons encouraging activities using colour and art work, reminding us that life changes just like the seasons, even if we don't want it to. Establishing trust and confidentiality is essential at this stage so the group can learn how to work effectively and with respect. Group rules are drawn up and kept as a focus throughout the programme. It is noted how respectful the children and young people are of the need to be aware of confidentiality. Group members really appreciate hearing how Companions have coped with loss in their lives, and this reinforces the sense of connectedness that is such an important feature of the programme.

By session seven, using the imagery of a kite, the children are asked to think of people they know and things they can do to help through difficult times, emphasizing that if a kite is unattached, it floats aimlessly. The tail provides balance and support, and the children are encouraged to make their kite stable and balanced through noting on the ribbons attached to the tail who and what is important and helps them to feel grounded. Throughout the eight sessions, the mutual sharing of experiences and strategies for coping bind the children and young people into ongoing peer support.

What primary school age children say about how Seasons' groups helped

- Handle your problems properly
- That things don't always go my way and I'm not the only one whose life has changed
- That it is not your fault what happens
- It is OK to feel sad or upset sometimes but don't take it out on other people
- To be confident with my self
- That I can change my life around
- When I'm upset, I could go and talk to someone about it or do something which I like doing.

The following edited transcript of a conversation with three teenage girls, reflecting on their experience of a Seasons for Growth group, gives a flavour of the process and the social, emotional, and spiritual outcomes for the teenagers.

Q What has been helpful about being in a group?

A Well, it's helpful because you can talk to people. Because it's easier to know how other people are feeling because you feel like when somebody has died, that if you feel that it's just you who have to cope with the situation but it's not. It's other people as well. Sometimes you can't talk to people and you feel that if somebody starts it off, you can just talk. It helps.

Q How would you like friends to be towards you?

A Supportive. Very supportive. Because you haven't really got anybody to support you going through what you're going through. So it's easier to come here where you can talk to people but friends, they don't understand. They say: 'Oh I'm sorry about that'. But you want somebody that can talk to you about what you're going through. Like to say: 'How are you doing today?' And 'How's this?' That really helps.

B No, I hate people feeling sorry for me.

A No, but it helps when people say 'How are you feeling?' 'How are you today?' and 'How has it been?' It makes you forget really about your hurting.

Q **What's it like on really bad days?**

A On really, really bad days, it's terrible. You just feel like it's the end of the world really. You feel ….

B Rubbish. To put it in polite terms.

A You feel like killing yourself sometimes. Because sometimes people just don't listen to you, and sometimes people shout at you and that makes you angrier. I know that sounds a bit selfish. But people shout at you, but you feel totally like nobody's really there for you.

B Like my foster parent. She starts shouting, then I start shouting at her, and then we need to start sitting down and talking as if nothing's wrong. Like the minute you walked in the door you knew there was something wrong with me.

A My school's really been supportive, but sometimes teachers, don't really know what you're going through. Like if it's supply teachers. 'Oh, write about your Mum, write about your Dad'. And all that. But you go: 'I'm not comfortable about writing about my Mum and my Dad. I don't really know you. I don't really want to share my details and stuff with you'. So it's hard as well.

Q **So can you say how long it's been since your Mum died and how are you feeling now?**

A Because they died at the same, like nearly, about a year apart, so it's a lot easier for us now than it was then, because it was like my Mum died and then it was my Da and then it was: 'Oh God, this is too fast for me, it's just going too fast'. But as the days go by, it gets easier and sometimes you just feel that nobody cares and you can be pulled down, and then other days you can feel quite happy. It's just the way your mood is and the way it changes. You feel a bit selfish for it, but it happens.

Q **Do you still talk to your Mum and Dad?**

B I write letters and then I put them in the fire, so they're like going in the air.

A I never thought of that. That's nice. I always talk to my Ma. Every time I get in my bed. I say: 'Oh I done this today, I done that'. And I feel to myself, can she hear me? And sometimes I think she can, hopefully.

Helping the family

Parents and carers are invited to learn about the group process and in some agencies the Adult Component of the programme (additional training required) is run in parallel sessions, thus opening up communication within families. Parents reflecting on their children's experience commented:

What were the best aspects of the programme for your child?

+ The confidence, understanding, and ability to relate to other children that she has gained have allowed my child to speak more openly. She now realises she has choices and can act accordingly and can communicate well how she feels.

+ I feel he has come out of his shell; his confidence has come on amazing.

+ My child seems to be less frustrated and angry; she expresses feelings in words more than temper and frustration.

The most challenging aspects?

+ Taking on board compliments from others.

+ The ability to speak openly, to have the confidence to speak to other people regarding issues and feelings.

The most important learning?

+ To know that things happen within families, and it's ok to experience a variety of feelings regardless of what they are, and to deal with it and move on.

+ That she can trust other people within the group. Learning how to deal with her feelings. Creating friendships with others.

Support for Companions: developing a network

Regular Reconnectors, arranged by Seasons Trainers, support Companions ensuring adherence to the core elements of the programme, sharing good practice and encouraging communities in the support of emotionally vulnerable children. Following a very supportive experience of the programme five years ago in primary school, a group of young people have taken part in a film to promote Seasons for Growth. Two national conferences have taken place to give Companions new ideas for working with emotionally vulnerable children and promoting a strong sense of commitment to the Seasons programme. In Scotland a National Co-ordinator post has been funded by the Scottish Government to promote awareness and co-ordinate support for Companions.

In summary, the rationale for Seasons for Growth is based on the belief that grief is normal and can be a valuable part of life. Children and adolescents need to be provided with the opportunity to examine how grief as a result of death, separation, or divorce has impacted their lives. The bonus is that children also gain confidence from helping others.

References

Brown, D. (2007) Childhood Bereavement *Elementary Scottish Journal of Healthcare Chaplaincy,* **1**(2): 28–31.

Hamera, A. et al. (2008) Non-standard families and the role of the EP. *Educational Psychology in Scotland,* **10**(1): 8–13.

Klass, D. (1999) *The Spiritual Lives of Bereaved Parents.* New York: Brunner-Mazel Inc.

Stroebe, M. and Schut, H. (1999) The dual process model of coping with bereavement. *Death Studies,* **23**, 197–224.

Worden, J.W. (1996) *Children and Grief: When a Parent Dies.* New York: Guildford.

Choose Life http://www.chooselife.net (accessed 7th January 2009).

Good Grief Australia http://www.goodgrief.org.au (accessed 7th January 2009).

Seasons for Growth contacts

Notre Dame Centre (Scotland)
http://www.notredamecentre.org.uk (accessed 7th January 2009)
http://www.seasonsforgrowth.org.uk (accessed 7th January 2009)
England and Wales
http://www.seasonsforgrowth.co.uk (accessed 7th January 2009)

Chapter 14

Working with volunteers to provide bereavement support to children

Rosie Nicol-Harper

'I enjoy being a friendly face, who is there, solely, for that child or young person'.

'It is a delight to see a child's pleasure in creating something beautiful to evoke memories of a parent, and there is immense satisfaction in helping him communicate his bottled up emotions so that he can deal with them'.

'The opportunity to work with young people, to feel that it is possible to make a difference'.

This is what three new volunteers in a child bereavement service said when they were asked what they enjoy most about the work.

This chapter aims to highlight some of the issues, challenges, and joys encountered when using volunteers to provide bereavement support to children. It draws on the literature available and the practical experience gained by one organization, which was founded around the use of volunteers to provide face-to-face support to young people. The chapter aims to show that there is no 'one size fits all' policy for using volunteers whilst emphasizing the richness that volunteers bring. Although child bereavement services may use volunteers in a number of ways, including administration or fundraising, this chapter focuses on using volunteers directly providing bereavement support to children.

What do we mean by volunteers providing bereavement support?

Historically, volunteers have played a major role in the provision of adult bereavement support, both generically and within the field of palliative care. Colin Murray Parkes has suggested that 'When we consider the skills that are needed, the ability to provide reassurance, emotional support, and the kind of security that we associate with good parenting; it may be that carefully selected, trained and supported volunteers are sometimes better than clever professionals whose paper qualifications may outweigh their ability to handle human relationships with sensitivity and tact'. (Parkes 2006 p267)

A recent survey of UK childhood bereavement services, conducted in 2000, found that 87% of services were reliant to some degree on unpaid staffing, with 14% being entirely dependent on unpaid staff (Rolls and Payne 2003). Of these volunteers, 91% had direct contact with children and/or parents (Rolls and Payne 2008).

In many cases, volunteers provide grief support as opposed to bereavement counselling.

An in-depth study of volunteers based in a well-established palliative care service, providing a direct service to bereaved adults, found that bereaved adults valued being listened to, feeling understood, having support from someone outside their social network and receiving reassurance about common grief experiences (Relf 2000). Relf summarizes the advantages of volunteer support for bereaved people as follows:

+ The involvement of volunteers reinforces that grief is a natural response and not an illness
+ Volunteer support may be perceived as less distant and less threatening than professional therapy
+ Volunteers have the potential to educate and influence others in the community about loss and bereavement
+ Volunteers understand and represent their community in a way that professionals alone cannot.

These final two points may be particularly pertinent issues for children's bereavement services, where public education about the needs of bereaved children and the need to seek ongoing financial support from the communities they serve are critical.

Clarifying the role of volunteers in an organization

Using volunteers requires clarity of thinking by the organization about exactly what the volunteer's role is to be. The format of recruitment, selection, training, and supervision of volunteers is entirely dependent on their specific role. For example, someone who volunteers to assist supervised group activities once or twice per year will require different training and ongoing supervision from someone who will be offering direct one-to-one support to a child over a period of time within the child's home, or from someone providing office-based telephone support.

The needs of the organization, the clients, and the volunteers all have to be taken into account. For a service offering direct one-to-one bereavement support to children, we believe that these include the following points:

The needs of the organization

The organization needs:

- ◆ Volunteers who show commitment – to training; to the work; to the children and families
- ◆ Volunteers who are mentally robust, who can tolerate, and not be frightened by, strong feelings
- ◆ Volunteers who are willing to reflect on their own loss, and who have a belief in the ability of the client to build on inner strength and to grow through the experience of bereavement
- ◆ Volunteers who can treat each client as an individual and not be tied to fixed expectations about the duration or frequency of their need for support
- ◆ Volunteers who can realistically fulfil the time commitment
- ◆ Volunteers with strong and flexible personal support via family and friends
- ◆ Volunteers who can continue to learn, grow, and add to the service.

The needs of the clients

The clients need someone:

- ◆ who is sensitive to their needs
- ◆ who is trustworthy, reliable, and predictable
- ◆ who is open to learning about the different ways that children grieve and how best they can be supported
- ◆ who can stay with them through difficult emotional experiences without panicking or trying to move them away from difficult feelings
- ◆ who can be flexible, and who is not tied to their own agenda.

The needs of the volunteer

The volunteers need:

- ◆ To feel supported
- ◆ To feel a valued part of a team

- Opportunities to gain experience and to learn new skills
- To be able to identify with the aims and ethos of the organization and to feel connected to it
- To feel that they can make a difference and offer a unique contribution that will be recognized and celebrated.

The implications of using volunteers

On a practical level, an organization's commitment to its volunteers is demonstrated by clear and accessible policies and procedures. These include: equal opportunities policy guiding recruitment procedures; clarity about the need for Criminal Records Bureau checks; a volunteer management policy which links to explicit problem-solving procedures; a system of supervision and periodic appraisal or review. Training will also be required to explain the organization's safeguarding children policy; health and safety guidelines, especially in relation to home visiting and lone working; data protection and record-keeping policy. Detailed service development guides covering areas to consider are available through the Childhood Bereavement Network. Systems and paperwork should be developed to monitor the activity of volunteers. Recording the hours they are donating is just as important as being able to claim their agreed expenses, such as travel, phone calls, or materials used with clients. It serves as a very practical way of demonstrating that the organization recognizes and values their time and contribution. A helpful guide to the importance of good volunteer management is provided by the National Council for Voluntary Organisations (2008).

It is a common misconception that using volunteers means that no costs are involved. Using volunteers to provide direct support can be very cost-effective, but budgets should include costs associated with recruitment and selection, training and induction, insurance, travel and other expenses, supervision, and social events. There are also some 'hidden' organizational costs to consider:

- Introducing volunteers into an existing service may leave paid staff feeling threatened, over-cautious, anxious, or even hostile about the capabilities of volunteers. Time to carefully prepare all personnel involved and clarity about the respective roles is essential
- Staff may not have the relevant expertise or confidence to provide training
- Staff time to organize and deliver training to volunteers may compromise the core functions of the organization in the short term. If training and support sessions for volunteers take place in the evenings or weekends, time off during the week for staff will be necessary
- Ongoing staff time with volunteers is often underestimated, especially during the early stages of volunteering, when they may need frequent, regular access.

SeeSaw's approach to working with volunteers to provide bereavement support to children

Background to SeeSaw's service

From the outset, SeeSaw was a collaborative project. Health professionals responsible for adult bereavement support at Sir Michael Sobell House, a palliative care unit in Oxford, England, together with a child psychiatrist and other local children's professionals, identified the lack of co-ordinated provision for the special grief support needs of children.

SeeSaw was established in 1999 as a registered charity to provide 'grief support to the young of Oxfordshire'. It was staffed with a Director charged with setting up a service based around using volunteers to provide individualized support to young people. A small paid team (2.8 full time equivalents) provided essential administration and fundraising functions alongside a support service to professionals, with a particular emphasis on schools. This has been supplemented by a full-time pre-bereavement worker and a further team member to manage increased referrals and develop groupwork. In total, 45 volunteers have been trained and 13 currently operate as volunteer support workers.

Although local health, social care, and education professionals promote the service to parents of bereaved children, all client families are self-referred. As Oxfordshire is a large, mainly rural county, albeit with urban pockets of economic deprivation, the model of support is based around home visiting to ensure the service is accessible to all who need it.

When appropriate, following a home assessment of each family's needs by members of the staff team, support workers meet with children at home, or occasionally in the SeeSaw family room, or in a child's school. There is no set way of providing support – much will depend on the child's age, understanding, and needs. Sometimes the best support is by meeting with or regularly phoning a parent rather than a child, so support workers need to be very flexible.

Seesaw's recruitment, selection, and training of volunteer support workers

This section covers what has been termed the ABC of using volunteers: Acquiring, Building, and Cherishing them (Osborne 1999).

Acquiring volunteers – recruitment and selection

The aim of each cycle of recruitment is to ensure that as many people with the right attributes and availability learn about the need for volunteers, whilst making sure the organization's efforts and resources are targeted as effectively as possible. We have found:

- A broad approach to advertising is most effective, using articles in village newsletters, flyers on local government and health service staff noticeboards and other local websites, news items on local radio stations, and targeted newspaper adverts

- A strategy is needed to explain alternative forms of volunteering, such as fundraising or administrative help, to those responders who cannot proceed to training

- Taster evenings explain the training programme in some depth. Staff members and an existing support worker talk about their roles, a video is shown of bereaved children talking about their experiences, and the selection process and training programme is described. We also incorporate a brief exercise, i.e. talking in pairs about a childhood loss, not only to give a flavour of the nature of the training, but also to assess an applicant's ability to be part of a learning group and to tolerate sharing information about themselves

- In light of the experiential nature of the training course, it is not suitable for anyone who has experienced a major bereavement within the past two years. This is reiterated as a 'health warning' at the outset of the taster evening, as some people who have recently experienced grief may feel especially drawn to this area of volunteering

- We are very clear about the level of commitment needed to become a volunteer support worker for SeeSaw. On average, the regular commitment is 16 hours per month (including meetings and supervision), for a period of two years or more

- Applicants need to be available in late afternoons or early evenings as this is when contact time with families and meetings usually take place. This may prove particularly difficult for people with school age children

- Recruiting volunteers with specific skills such as leading a one-off drama workshop, or recruiting volunteers to co-run activity days, or groups for bereaved parents may require a different approach to the model described here

- Having received all the above information, interested persons complete an application form. We have found it helpful to ask applicants open-ended questions in their application form such as 'What aspects of your childhood and adolescence did you like (and dislike) particularly?' These give an indication to the applicant of the importance we place on self-awareness and are helpful starting points for discussion at interview

- We have a formal interview process. Not all applicants are necessarily short-listed for interview
- We build in enough time so that references can be taken up before interview for those shortlisted. Referees are specifically asked to comment on an applicant's mental and emotional robustness, and their ability to listen to families in distress with non-judgemental warmth.

Building volunteers – initial training

SeeSaw's volunteer support worker training course is made up of about 40 teaching hours. The course content covers three major elements:

1 **Personal Content** – *for participants to*:
   - develop a better understanding of their own experience of loss
   - explore personal anxieties of loss through death
   - develop an understanding of loss using their own experience as a baseline.

2 **Theory** – *for participants to*:
   - become familiar with the theoretical understanding of bereavement
   - understand how a child's developmental age and stage influences their experience of loss
   - understand the context of support work e.g. family systems, schools, etc.
   - understand how to work safely following safeguarding children policy guidelines.

3 **Practical Experience** – *for participants to*:
   - develop basic listening skills within a context of bereavement support
   - recognize the limits of the service SeeSaw can offer and to understand when to refer on
   - develop practical skills that will enhance the delivery of bereavement support.

In addition to the time commitment for attendance, approximately 20 hours is needed for guided background reading, writing a learning journal, and project making. As the course programme builds on each previous session, and to maintain good group dynamics if anyone misses more than two sessions, they are unable to continue the training course.

Cherishing volunteers – supervision, on-going training, and review

At the heart of an effective and safe service for children is regular, dependable and thorough supervision with review. This ensures not only the consistency and accountability of the service – 'quality control' – but also ensures that the work is not having a detrimental effect on the individual. Small and large group supervision are seen as essential requirements of working with SeeSaw. In the rare instances where volunteers have been unable to maintain this commitment, we have either agreed a period of leave of absence, or reached a decision for the volunteer to leave the service.

Small group supervision

- We provide monthly supervision to volunteers in small groups of two, three, or four. Having a group larger than four prevents having adequate time for each person to share their current work
- As peer learning is such an important element of small group supervision, each group is carefully selected to include members with a range of experience, length of service, and interests
- The groups are facilitated by clinicians experienced in working with children. We have found that it is important that group supervisors understand the importance of bolstering the confidence of volunteers, perhaps drawing out their experience and competence in other aspects of their lives, whilst still being able to appropriately challenge and guide individuals' practice and facilitate peer group learning
- Regular supervisors' meetings are held to ensure clear communication between the supervisors and the director, who retains clinical responsibility for the service provided by the volunteers.

Large group supervision and ongoing training

- Large group supervision and training takes place monthly. Meetings include an eclectic mix of practical refresher training, case discussions, advancing knowledge of theoretical topics, and information about the organization's activities
- One meeting a year takes place at a weekend in order to cover a topic in greater depth
- Two meetings a year are specifically social events and also provide an opportunity for Trustees to meet volunteers and reinforce how much their unique contribution is valued.

Annual review

An annual review is provided to:

- provide a mutual opportunity to reflect back and comment on the past year's achievements or challenges

- consider the cumulative impact of the work on the volunteer
- consider the impact of the work on a volunteer's support networks
- reassess what areas of work they may now feel confident to take on
- review training needs
- seek feedback on communication and supervision structures.

For maximum objectivity, the review is completed by someone other than the volunteer's supervisor. Comments gained through this process have over the years been invaluable in influencing how SeeSaw's service has developed.

Who volunteers?

A UK survey of childhood bereavement services found that the majority of unpaid staff respondents (n = 65 or 88%) were female (Rolls and Payne 2008). Currently SeeSaw has no male support workers and only a handful of men have applied to be trained. We have a mixture of volunteers in full or part-time employment, while some are retired or not working. The age and gender distribution of our volunteers is skewed by the level of availability we require. However, a groupwork programme might seek volunteers who could commit to several weekends a year, and therefore successfully recruit more men and younger adults.

Many of our volunteers are professionally qualified in areas of childcare or adult care, e.g. health visiting, social work, teaching, or counselling, but this is not a prerequisite. In some instances it has been harder to 'unlearn' a professional role or style in order to provide appropriate grief support than for other volunteers without such a background. For this reason and for practical and time considerations, we have a policy of not normally considering anyone for our training who is still completing a training in another field. Other child bereavement organizations with a counselling or other therapeutic focus may offer training placements when resources for supervision allow, and where there is an overall fit with the organization's objectives and methods.

Lessons learned

Over the years, our recruitment, training, and support of volunteers has needed to be adapted. Specifically:

- We have learned to be explicit that the training is designed to equip people with the skills and confidence to become SeeSaw support workers rather than to be a general child bereavement training
- We found that where volunteers themselves have school age children, they often only completed a short period of volunteering. We now stress the

likely practical difficulties and impact on the volunteer (and their support network, especially a partner) and only rarely accept someone with children onto the training

◆ Introducing a mid-term training interview allows for any concerns to be explored and time for these to be addressed through additional skills practice

◆ We have recruited staff who have experience of adult learning and training in addition to their child bereavement skills

◆ As most of their visits take place outside office hours, volunteers are provided with the home contact details of the Director and all supervisors so that they can seek advice and support whenever they need it. It has only been required very occasionally, but it is provided in recognition of the solitary, and potentially isolating, nature of their task, and the need to safeguard those children receiving a service

◆ The social element of small and large group supervision has been found to be a significantly important part of fostering group identity and ensuring each volunteer feels part of something both worthwhile but also enjoyable.

The combined findings of studies exploring young people's wishes for help from support systems found that the main rule was for flexibility (Dyregrov and Dyregrov 2008 p92). We have found that using volunteers massively increases our ability to offer a flexible service for the following reasons:

◆ There are limited times when children are free and not too tired, so having volunteers available at those times means that many more children can be seen without them needing to miss part of their school day. For bereaved children already struggling with 'feeling different' it can be a great relief that they do not need to come out of class and then have to explain to curious peers where they've been

◆ For a home-based service, using volunteers ensures that the limited travelling time of any paid staff can be directed where most needed

◆ Giving a few hours per week dilutes the exposure to suffering and loss, and means that the volunteers are unlikely to get saturated with grief

◆ Volunteers' enthusiasm for their role is likely to generate awareness of the service, especially within their own communities, and to generate goodwill with a potentially wider pool of personal contacts

◆ Sharing their wide variety of different life experiences, skills, and motivations, volunteers often generate new and exciting ideas. This richness, creativity and enthusiasm can have real benefits for clients but also for paid staff, who can enjoy co-creating resources or to be re-energized in their own direct work.

Having described some of the challenges and advantages of using volunteers, the last words belong to a parent who has had first-hand experience.

'Thank you for sending us (volunteer name). She helped my daughter to have some-one she could talk to about the death of her sister without getting upset, and to make her feel special. She gave her the one-to-one that had disappeared as I was struggling so much. It gave me and my partner time to open up to each other and recognize the issues we needed to work through. Our volunteer was my safety net. She helped us immensely and we are eternally grateful. I would like her to know how strong we feel. My child says: "It was very fun and it made me feel happier". Thank you'.

References

Childhood Bereavement Network *Service Development Guides* Available at: http://www.childhoodbereavementnetwork.org.uk/policyPractice_service.htm (accessed 25 November 2008).

Dyregrov, K. and Dyregrov, A. (2008) *Effective Grief and Bereavement Support. The Role of Family, Friends, Colleagues, Schools and Support Professionals.* London: Jessica Kingsley Publishers.

National Council for Voluntary Organisations *Volunteer Management Policies.* Available at: http://www.volunteering.org.uk/resources/goodpracticebank. (Accessed 1 September 2009).

Osborne, C. (1999) The ABC's of bereavement volunteers: Acquire, build, cherish. *American Journal of Hospice and Palliative Care*, 380–385 quoted in Rolls, L. and Payne, S.A. (2008).

Parkes, C.M. (2006) *Love and Loss: The Roots of Grief and its Complications.* Hove: Routledge.

Relf, M. (2000) *The Effectiveness of Volunteer Bereavement Care: An Evaluation of a Palliative Care Bereavement Service.* Unpublished thesis, Goldsmiths, University of London.

Rolls, L. and Payne, S. (2003) Childhood bereavement services: A survey of UK provision. *Palliative Medicine*, 17: 423–432.

Rolls, L. and Payne, S. (2008) The voluntary contribution to UK childhood bereavement services: Locating the place and experiences of unpaid staff. *Mortality*, 13: 258–281.

Chapter 15

Brief interventions in critical care environments

Peter Speck[*]

Introduction

Family structures and attitudes regarding children and death have changed enormously over the past 100 years. Victorian art frequently depicts children involved in death bed scenes and the funeral processions. In recent times, however, there is a tendency to be protective of young children, to shield them from the reality of death, seeing the body, and sometimes from the funeral itself. The consequences of such 'protectiveness' can be far reaching for some people and lay the foundations for a variety of problems in later life, especially if the death is sudden and unexpected.

Even 50 years ago little work had been done to try to understand the effect of loss on young children. Health professionals frequently perceived the hospitalized, withdrawn child patient as compliant and 'content' and while the work of Robertson (1952) was initially received with scepticism, it did indicate that the young child's quietness was often an indication of traumatization. Staff training seemed to contain little understanding of the impact of death on the young child.

Over the years, attitudes within society have changed. Research has increased our knowledge of the way in which children develop their understanding of the concept of death. Pioneer figures include Bowlby (1969), Wolfenstein (1966) Furman (1974) and Caplan (1969). In more recent years the work of Parkes (1996), Worden (2003), Stroebe (1993), Black (1978), and others has extended our understanding of how people seek to adjust to major losses in their life, and drawn attention to the needs of young children and siblings. Current understanding indicates that children need immediate and honest answers that allow them to share in the family grief. They need to know the truth communicated with warmth. If children's questions and feelings are postponed or ignored by the adults around, then these children may conclude

---

[*] Former healthcare chaplain. Visiting Fellow, Faculty of medicine, Southampton University.

that they may be responsible in some way, or that their feelings are unacceptable, and push them underground.

Current research findings have not always filtered through to the general population. In my role as a healthcare chaplain, I frequently needed to enquire of parents and families whether they had thought about what to say to the children following a traumatic death of a baby, older sibling, or adult. Not infrequently the response was 'they are too young to understand' or 'It would be too upsetting for them at their age' and we then began an exploration together of what the surviving child may already know, and what their needs might be. In this chapter we shall look at a small selection of situations where the needs of children have been addressed following sudden unexpected death in an acute hospital setting and highlight some of the key elements in trying to minimize the risk of a complicated grief outcome.

Pregnancy loss

Most Acute Trust hospitals in the UK will have developed policies, quality standards and designated members of staff who can offer advice and support to couples who are facing pregnancy loss. This may be because of miscarriage, termination of the foetus following diagnosis of genetic or other abnormality, or for non-therapeutic reasons. It may be towards the end of the pregnancy that complications occur and the mother has an intra-uterine death or the live baby is stillborn. In each of these situations there will be a varying degree of opportunity to prepare those most involved with the pregnancy. The work of self-help groups such as SANDS (stillbirth and neonatal death society) have had a key role to play in helping professional healthcare staff to assess sensitively the needs of the family, enable them to address the reality of the event, create appropriate memorialization, and obtain ongoing support as appropriate. The siblings of the unborn child often have knowledge of the impending arrival of a new brother or sister and may well have experienced natural sibling rivalry. This may not be mentionable to parents, especially if the parents are distressed about the actual or impending loss. If the death of the baby is not referred to, young children can be left wondering if their rivalrous thoughts have been powerful enough to kill the baby. Distinguishing reality from phantasy can be difficult even for older children let alone the very young. It is therefore important that there is some exploration with the mother (and father) about what the other children may already know and feel about the new baby and the mother's admission to hospital. This exploration needs to extend to include those siblings without demanding too much of them.

If the loss has not yet occurred there can be discussion of attitudes and feelings regarding seeing the dead foetus/baby. There is a difference between 'providing opportunity' and implying an 'ought to do'. This relates to viewing, photographs, attending funerals, creating memory boxes, etc. It is especially important to be sensitive to cultural issues which may not always match a more general expectation based on the family's religious affiliation. A family from Nigeria, who happen to be Christian, may want nothing to do with the dead child because, as one father told me, 'We have nothing to do with dead babies. They are simply passing through here and we let them go'. To encourage a mother to see, touch and photograph her dead baby might, therefore, be encouraging her to go against the cultural norms of her family.

Many parents recognize the significance of giving their other children opportunity to be involved as far as they wish. It is important that the children are prepared for what they will see as many will never have seen a dead person of any age. Bringing the baby, suitably dressed and wrapped, into the mother's room in a 'Moses' basket or cot is more natural. The mother may then take the child into her arms and the sibling look at the child or perhaps take over the holding of the baby. Talking about the death and the reasons (where known) in a clear and simple way is also important. A member of staff, such as counsellor, midwife, or healthcare chaplain should be present to 'hold the boundaries' and free the parents to be distressed. The other adult can then be there for the sibling.

Avoid euphemisms and use clear terms such as 'dead, died, was unable to continue growing inside mummy's tummy'. Frequently this viewing and examination of the dead baby leads to discussion of what happens to the body now. This may include a post-mortem examination. 'The doctors will wish to examine the baby carefully to see if they can discover why X or Y stopped growing etc'. 'Then you and your family will need to decide how you want to say goodbye to X or Y'. Depending on the age of the siblings, this may lead to discussion of burial, cremation, coffins, putting toys into the coffin, whether the younger children want, or should, attend. Sensitivity is required to avoid steering people into undertaking activities because 'we' believe they will be good for them. However, people must make informed choice based on realistic options.

Cot death

Many of the above points apply equally to the distressing arrival of a dead baby in the Accident and Emergency (A and E) department. The child may sometimes be accompanied by a child minder who discovered the baby 'blue' in its pram or cot, or by a distraught parent who has discovered the child dead late at night. In either case, there is the additional complication of a necessary police investigation and coroner's autopsy to ensure that the death is a sudden infant death and not the result of another person's action. The mutual blame that surrounds cot death for many couples is compounded by the necessary coroner's involvement. Sensitivity by the emergency services in undertaking their necessary roles frequently helps to alleviate some of the distress for the parents. Siblings may not always be involved at this early acute stage and may temporarily be cared for by other adults. However, at some point their feelings and reactions need to be listened to so that they can be given permission to grieve with the rest of the family and not be shut out. It may be that this is picked up by their having the opportunity to see the dead child in the hospital mortuary viewing room, the A and E department, or at the funeral directors.

Viewing

Case study

Two young children aged five and nine expressed the wish to see their dead baby brother (Mark) who had been stillborn at 26 weeks gestation. The parents thought the nine-year old boy would cope but were not so sure about his sister. In talking with the five-year old she was adamant.'I know mummy was having a new baby. She's crying because Mark is dead and I want to say goodnight'. It was agreed that chaplain, nurse, parents, and children would go to see the baby. The baby was dressed in a 'Babygro' and placed in a crib. We sat in the waiting area which was a comfortably furnished 'sitting room' environment and discussed what we would see. When the baby was brought to the family the nine-year old boy hung back, but the five-year old immediately came forward to have a good look. The parents were tearful and seemed unable to respond to the children. The chaplain pointed out features of the dead baby – the dark hair, the finger nails the nose similar to the little girl. She then said 'Can I touch Mark?' 'Yes', I said. 'Touch his face gently and hold his hand'. She did so and then touched the top of his head. 'It's all squishy', she exclaimed. 'That's because Mark's head has not grown properly. Now that he's dead the bones won't join up firmly'. She then touched her head and said 'My head's not squishy'. 'No', I replied, 'that's because you're alive and your head's all joined up'. She then turned to her brother, took his hand and led him across to the baby and said 'You feel'. He did so, somewhat apprehensively, and then grinned and touched his own head. Finally the little girl said 'Goodnight Mark' kissed him and then sat down, sucked her thumb, and hugged her mother. Gradually the rest of the family said their farewells and prepared to leave.

In many ways the five-year old led the way and 'managed' the event, but it was crucial that there were people there who could be with the parents and free them to grieve in the presence of the children, while other adults could be there specifically for the children. Honesty about the meaning of being alive and being dead in response to the discoveries by the child was important. A key element was being reasonably comfortable with death and dead bodies as a healthcare professional, together with a willingness to be flexible in response to the young child's wish to lead. Healthcare staff may feel diffident about encouraging or responding to questions from children about death and dying. Thompson and Payne (2000) indicate that children within the age range of six – fourteen years can have a variety of questions to which they would like answers. In particular they welcome a doctor answering 'how and why' people die. By valuing the child's questions, a doctor can enhance the child's self-esteem at a time when children can be feeling especially vulnerable and unable to explore these ideas with other adults who may be too distressed.

Sudden death following a road traffic collision

Case study

A family were returning from holiday along a dual carriageway. It was late at night and pouring with rain. In the car were a husband and wife and their three children – a girl (aged seven) and twin boys (aged five). At traffic lights the father failed to stop in time and drove into a small lorry crossing the junction. In the resultant crash the mother was seriously injured and was dead on arrival at the hospital. The father had serious injuries and was admitted to intensive care. One of the twin boys was dead at the scene, the other was injured and, in the Accident and Emergency department, his sister with a severe head injury was in the paediatric intensive care. The chaplain on call had been called to A and E to offer support and assistance.

Given that the father and surviving daughter were unconscious in intensive care, the main focus was the needs and responses of the surviving twin and any other family members. The parents of the wife who had died in the crash had been contacted by the police and were making the 120-mile journey to the hospital. Family Liaison Officers (FLOs) had been assigned to the various people involved in the incident. Their assistance and support over the days and weeks that followed proved to be invaluable (see Capter 18). The surviving five-year old twin was in pain from several fractures but was becoming more responsive and beginning to ask for his mother. The child (Tom) knew there had been a crash and a big bang, but asked no questions and volunteered no information. It was explained that mummy had been involved in the crash with him and was being looked after in another part of the hospital. The subject of the other family members was not raised at this time. The child's grandmother had relayed a message via the police that she would like to be there when Tom was told more details and it was agreed to wait, if possible, for their arrival.

On meeting it was clear there was a good relationship between the children and the grandparents. The chaplain, FLO, and A and E staff brought them up to date on the condition of the family survivors. In spite of her own shock and grief, the grandmother still wished to tell Tom about his mother and she and the chaplain rehearsed how that might be done. They also considered the pros and cons of giving or withholding the news of the other family members. It was decided that they would try to follow Tom's lead rather than push the agenda and risk overloading him. The grandmother also wished her husband and the chaplain to be there with her. The unit had a special paediatric section, and this was chosen as an appropriate setting as there were books, games and pictures to make the whole environment more child friendly.

Children, like adults, may respond in a variety of ways to news of sudden death: shock and disbelief 'I don't believe you. You're telling lies', or dismay and protest, 'Be quiet! Go away I hate you!' or withdrawal and apathy. The child will often look hurt and puzzled by what is happening but show no emotional response. The child may also quickly switch from the information to wanting to engage with normal activity 'Put the television on'. It is best if the news is given by a close relative or family member, but as in this case, supported by someone else who is not quite so emotionally involved or overwhelmed. Healthcare staff can themselves, of course, feel overwhelmed by identification with the situation and need support before, and debriefing opportunities after, such encounters. Again clear language is important and the information should be short and to the point. Amplification of the circumstances can come later in response to questions, or after a period of time to let the first statements sink in.

Case study

In the above case, after hugs and kisses from Grandmother she said, 'Tom, you know you were in a car crash today. I have some very sad and bad news for you. Mummy was badly hurt in the crash and she has died. That's why she isn't here with you now'. There was a stunned silence. Then Tom said, 'I WANT Mummy NOW'. To which granny replied, 'I know darling, but mummy died in the crash'. Tom then started to cry and the two of them cried together for a while. Tom then said 'Can I see mummy again?', and granny looked at the chaplain who said, 'When your body is a bit better and you can move around we could take you to see mummy's body if you still want to'. Tom then said to granny, 'Will you read me a story?'

It was after the story that Tom said, 'Where is daddy?' and it was explained that Daddy and Ruth were in a special part of the hospital having extra special treatment, and as soon as possible we would take him to see them. It was then that he mentioned his twin. Grandmother was clearly quite drained by this time and grandfather took over. He followed his wife's earlier lead and reminded Tom of the crash and mother's injuries and death, and then said that Tom's brother had also died in the crash. Tom said, 'Does that mean he's with mummy?' Granddad said, 'yes' and Tom replied, 'So he'll be alright then'.

At this point the chaplain left them together for a little, saying that he would be just outside, and reported back to the other key staff what had been happening – and sought personal support from the other team members. Then a member of the ambulance crew came into the unit with a small teddy bear. She had picked it up at the scene and thought it might belong to one of the surviving children. It turned out to be the dead twin's favourite bear, and over the ensuing weeks and months became an important transitional object for Tom and a link to his dead twin brother. The work commenced in the A and E department that evening was only a beginning and over the weeks that followed the family was kept together as far as possible. Their clinical needs made it difficult initially for them to be in the same unit but as soon as possible they were re-united and cared for in adjacent rooms.

Most Acute Trust hospitals have a Major Incident Response plan which links with that of the emergency services in the community. Part of that plan will usually include a psycho-social response team who will know, and trust, each other through training together and working together. This team will draw upon social work, psychology, psychiatry (adult and child), psychotherapy, bereavement counselling, and chaplaincy input. A major incident is officially 'declared' before the whole team swings into action. However, a crash, such as that described above, is a major incident for the family concerned and, as the de-briefing showed, can impact on a large number of people. In this instance the chaplain contacted the co-ordinator of the psycho-social response group, and together they identified the resources they would need to assess and respond to the needs of this family while they were in the hospital. It was recognized that the interventions that were possible at this point in their grief were important to minimize risk, but would need to lead to longer term care. The team also reviewed what resources might be available for on-going support after discharge home in terms of general support, or more specific referral to a trauma unit if required. One of the key roles for the chaplaincy in the ensuing weeks was helping the father (an atheist) to consider and plan the funerals. The final choice was a secular funeral, with burial in a woodland burial site near where the family took their holidays. The funerals were delayed for 10 weeks until all members of the family were well enough to attend. De-briefing was arranged for the A and E staff, the staff on the wards caring for family members, and the members of the emergency services involved at the crash scene (35 people attended). The ripple effect of such incidents, personally and professionally, was graphically demonstrated.

Death of an older child

Sudden death in the teenage years can happen for a variety of reasons. Commonly it follows trauma occasioned by road traffic accident, assault, murder, or suicide. It may also be the result of life threatening disease where the individual has received treatment and seems to be recovering and then suddenly collapses and dies. Occasionally the individual has an undiagnosed condition which spontaneously erupts leading to unexpected death.

In all these cases, the admission of the teenager to hospital, and usually intensive care, will also bring a variety of family and friends who will have a wide range of reactions to what has happened. Entering the waiting room of an intensive care unit to explain the likelihood of death, and to support this mixed group of people in their anticipatory grief, can be challenging. One of the most striking things is the recognition that there are various cultural norms operating and the needs of the parents and family members may be very different from those of the sub-culture to which the dying teenager belonged. In order to be sensitive to this, it is frequently necessary to separate out some of the groups, assess the needs, and establish a rapport with each group. A good level of co-operation and communication is required from the healthcare professional involved if the dynamics within and between the groups are to be contained and worked with in a positive way. Flexibility of response may also be called for, especially if there is a tendency to apportion blame regarding the lifestyle and influences upon the child who is dying.

Case study

Jan was a 17-year old girl attending sixth-form college in order to obtain 'A' level exams. Her work record had deteriorated and there were many arguments at home. She stayed out late at night and, at weekends, often staying overnight at friends. Her younger sister (aged 13 years) was not a confidante and so could shed little light on her lifestyle. Jan was binge drinking and experimenting with a variety of drugs at the weekend. One weekend her best friend had a bad experience and became very frightened. She asked Jan to go with her to Narcotics Anonymous (NA) and at the meeting Jan recognized herself. She attempted to follow the programme but not in any serious way. Her parents had no knowledge of this, and she was careful to hide her abuse from the family. One evening she took a lethal mix of drugs and collapsed in a night-club. The ambulance took her to the local hospital where, following admission to intensive care, she was put on a life-support machine. Her parents were contacted and arrived at the hospital, with Jan's sister, in a very distraught state. A number of Jan's friends also arrived – to mixed reception from the parents. Some were school friends who had some idea of Jan's recent habits, others were from the NA group. The clinical picture was poor and Jan had quickly gone into multi-organ failure. A first cycle of brain stem tests was performed and showed that Jan was virtually dead already. A further set would be undertaken the next day before decisions were made with the parents about ceasing life support. The social worker and chaplain assigned to intensive care agreed to work together, with the staff, with the parents, and Jan's peer group. This chapter focuses on the peer group rather than the parents, but clearly the parents' and sister's needs were paramount.

Thinking of the peer group in particular, it was important to try to establish the nature of the relationships and, with the parent's agreement, who should have access to Jan in what were to be her last hours. The parents, in spite of their emotional pain and ambivalence to some of the friends, were generous in allowing access to a group of about eight. Many of the youngsters were genuinely fond of Jan and deeply shocked at the turn of events. Most of them had no religious affiliation but felt in need of help in knowing what to do in the face of impending death. It was important first of all to establish that they were clear regarding the meaning of brain stem death and life support. It was explained that Jan's family were having to face saying goodbye to their daughter and had asked for help in doing that. Her friends might also feel the need for help in saying their goodbyes. Suggestions were made about touching or holding Jan, using her name, saying privately to her some of things they would like to say (or had said earlier), or saying out loud what they were feeling. They might like to have a brief period of time alone, or together, but they needed to be clear that this was a 'goodbye'. One of the group said that Jan had always wanted to swim with dolphins but had not been able to. Someone else phoned a brother and asked him to bring a CD of whale and dolphin sounds. With the parent's permission this was played by the bedside while the various youngsters came and sat or spoke to Jan. Towards the end of the evening, they understood that the remaining time was really for Jan's parents and family and it felt important to draw this little group together in some way. Acknowledging that a religious ritual was not appropriate for them, the chaplain suggested that they might like to listen or join in one prayer that he had brought with him. It was the 'serenity prayer' which is used at all NA and AA meetings.

> God grant me the serenity
> to accept the things I cannot change
> to change the things I can
> and the wisdom to know the difference.

All of them joined in and some spontaneously held hands as they did so. They then hugged Jan's parents and left the unit. The following morning the repeat neurological tests confirmed brain stem death and Jan's parents asked for life support to cease. The social worker and chaplain were present with the parents at the time Jan died, and the parents commented on how moving and supportive they had found the group of friends, in spite of their initial feelings of ambivalence and anger at their *assumed* role in Jan's life.

One of the key issues in this situation was working with the different people involved at different levels and, sometimes, as separate groups. Flexibility was also important on behalf of the health care professionals, the staff of the unit, and the chaplaincy, which might have been assumed to only be capable of responding in a religious way. Making sure that the clinical picture is clear is vital when there are issues regarding the withdrawal of life support as so many people find it hard to process what they know intellectually (that this person has already died – the brain stem has irreversibly ceased to function) from what they feel emotionally (the person cannot be dead because the body feels warm, the chest is moving up and down, and the heart is beating). Families need time for this processing, especially if the person dying is deemed a suitable candidate for organ donation. The tension between 'head' and 'heart' can be great and different family members and siblings can be at very different points in assimilating what is happening. Clear communication in a compassionate but straight-forward way is crucial. There needs to be relatively good and easy access to the dying person, with overnight accommodation available nearby. Most modern units have addressed these issues in both the design of the unit and the training of staff. Managing oneself in role can be easy or difficult for the healthcare professional depending on the circumstances surrounding the death. Sometimes there are a variety of unconscious 'hooks' which can draw the staff member in to an inappropriate level of involvement leading to feeling overwhelmed or actively 'sucked out' of role and ineffective (Speck 1987).

Recognizing one's limitations and being able to hand over to a colleague from the same, or a different, discipline can be an important strength. Staff support should be a regular part of the life of units which deal with trauma since you can never predict the cases which will draw you in more than others. Identification with the situation or persons involved in the event can be very powerful and unexpected. The fact that many of Jan's peer group were almost adult can also hide the fact that this may be the first close encounter with death for many and can trigger off a degree of regression in their behaviour and ability to cope. If offered in the right way, much good learning can occur at such times, which may strengthen their own coping repertoire for the future.

Summary

- Children do grieve if adults can recognize this and give them permission.
- Adults frequently deny the child's grief as a way of protecting the child and themselves from further pain.
- Children commonly mask their grief and also seek to protect the adult.
- The experience and expression of their grief is specifically linked to the child's emotional development and cultural patterns within the family and peer group.
- It is helpful to explore the child's fantasies and magical thinking since these can be sources of guilt and feelings of responsibility for the death
- A child's grief may be expressed indirectly through altered behaviour
- It is important to respond immediately to the child's grief, accepting their feelings and questions, whatever they may be, with open, honest answers
- Children should be involved as far as possible in the grief of the family, the reality of the death and the funeral.

Healthcare professionals

Involved in the care of children involved with the sudden death of an adult or sibling need to offer care that is individualized to that child and family, sensitive to the culture and beliefs of that family, and informed as to need for the child's own grief to be valued and expressed without coercion or collusion.

Above all it is helpful for professionals to remember the words of Bremner (2000).

'Young people are resilient and do grow and develop creatively if their experiences are acknowledged, their feelings respected and their questions about death and loss answered. However, with this age group (*she writes of adolescents*) more than any other, the professional has to have the most courage and least anxiety about getting it wrong. No matter how risky or uncomfortable it feels to us, almost any attempt to communicate and involve the young person is better than exclusion and silence'.

References

Black, D. (1978) The bereaved child. *Child Psychology,* **19**, 287–292.

Bowlby, J. (1969) *Attachment and Loss. Vol. I, Attachment.* London: Hogarth Press.

Bremner, I. (2000) Working with adolescents. *Bereavement Care,* **19**(1): 6–8.

Caplan, G. (1969) *An Approach to Community Mental Health.* London: Tavistock Publications.

Furman, E. (1974) *A Child's Parent Dies.* New Haven, CT: Yale University Press.

Lansdown, R., Frangoulis, S. and Jordan, N. (1997) Children's concept of an afterlife. *Bereavement Care,* **16**(2): 16–18.

Parkes, C.M. (1996) *Bereavement: Studies in Adult Life.* 3rd ed. London: Tavistock.

Robertson, J. (1952) Film *A Two Year Old Goes to Hospital.* Tavistock Child Dev. Res. Unit.

Speck, P. (1987) Working with dying people. In Obholtzer, A., Roberts, V. (eds) *The Unconscious at Work: Individual and Organizational Stress in the Human Services.* London: Routledge. pp. 94–100.

Stroebe, M., Stroebe, W. and Hansson, R. (1993) *Handbook of Bereavement: Theory, Research and Intervention.* Cambridge: Cambridge University Press.

Thompson, F. and Payne, S. (2000) Bereaved children's questions to a doctor. *Mortality,* 5(1): 74–96.

Wolfenstein, M. (1966) How is mourning possible? *Psycholanalytic Study of the Child,* **21**: 93.

Worden, J.W. (2003) *Grief Counselling and Grief Therapy.* 3rd ed. London: Brunner-Routledge.

Chapter 16

Working with traumatically bereaved children

William Yule and Patrick Smith

Introduction

Bereavement is part of normal human experience. It is often distressing, and some would say 'traumatic'. For a child to lose a parent or sibling can radically affect their life. But some deaths are truly traumatic – sudden, unexpected deaths; accidental deaths where the child witnesses the accident; murders where the child witnesses one parent killing another. In these circumstances, the child may develop particular stress reactions and depression as well as bereavement, and additional techniques may be required to help the child cope.

Elsewhere in this book, it is argued that the social support from family and friends is one of the most important factors in 'buffering' a child against any adverse effects of a bereavement. Being able to discuss the dead person, and their feelings for the deceased in a supportive way, is a normal, healthy part of coming to terms with a loss. But when that loss also may have affected the very support systems, then normal healing processes can be interrupted. When the supportive parent is no longer there, when the wider community has been devastated by a disaster, when the incident that caused the death is a horrific accident, then also the wider support systems may be unavailable or dysfunctional.

In such circumstances, the normal processes of grief and mourning may be affected by the experience of trauma. It is a widely held belief that grieving may be inhibited by the stress reactions and that these need to be treated first. As always, there are exceptions to any rule, but this advice seems to hold in general.

So what are these 'traumatic stress reactions' and how can they be treated so as to permit normal grieving to take place?

Traumatic stress reactions in children

Immediately following a very frightening experience, children are likely to be very distressed, tearful, frightened, and in shock. They need protection and safety. They need to be reunited with their families wherever possible.

Starting almost immediately, most children are troubled by *repetitive, intrusive thoughts* about the accident. Such thoughts can occur at any time, but particularly when the children are otherwise quiet, as when they are trying to drop off to sleep. At other times, the thoughts and vivid recollections are triggered off by reminders in their environment. A few children do experience *flashbacks* and report that they are re-experiencing the event as if it were happening all over again, but this is uncommon. *Sleep disturbances* are very common, particularly in the first few weeks. *Fears* of the dark and bad dreams, *nightmares*, and waking through the night are widespread (and often manifest outside the developmental age range in which they normally occur).

Separation difficulties are frequent, even among teenagers. For the first few days, children may not want to let their parents out of their sight, even reverting to sleeping in the parental bed. Many children become much more *irritable and angry* than previously, both with parents and peers.

Although child survivors experience a *pressure to talk* about their experiences, paradoxically they also find it very *difficult to talk with their parents and peers*. Often they do not want to upset the adults, and so parents may not be aware of the full extent of their children's suffering. Peers may hold back from asking what happened in case they upset the child further; the survivor often feels this as a rejection.

Children report a number of *cognitive changes*. Many experience *difficulties in concentration*, especially in school work. Others report *memory problems*, both in mastering new material and in remembering old skills such as reading music. They become very *alert to danger* in their environment, being adversely affected by reports of other disasters.

Survivors have learned that life is very fragile. This can lead to a loss of faith in the future or a *sense of foreshortened future*. Their priorities change. Some feel they should live each day to the full and not plan far ahead. Others realise they have been over-concerned with materialistic or petty matters and resolve to rethink their values. Their 'assumptive world' has been challenged (Janoff-Bulman 1985).

Not surprisingly, many develop *fears* associated with specific aspects of their experiences. They avoid situations they associate with the disaster. Many experience *survivor guilt* – about surviving when others died; about thinking they should have done more to help others; about what they themselves did to survive.

Adolescent survivors report significantly high rates of *depression*, some becoming clinically depressed, having suicidal thoughts, and taking overdoses in the year after a disaster. A significant number become very *anxious* after accidents, although the appearance of *panic attacks* is sometimes considerably delayed.

In summary, children and adolescents surviving a traumatic event show a wide range of symptoms, which tend to cluster around signs of re-experiencing the traumatic event, trying to avoid dealing with these intrusive memories and the emotions that they gives rise to, and a range of signs of increased physiological arousal. There may be considerable co-morbidity with depression, generalized anxiety or pathological grief reactions (Meiser-Stedman, 2002).

Post traumatic stress disorder – PTSD

Sometimes, these reactions may be both severe and prolonged. Indeed, they may interfere with normal adjustment and development to such an extent that the reaction warrants being diagnosed as a post traumatic stress disorder or PTSD. This is a particular pattern of symptoms in three clusters – intrusive thoughts and images about the traumatic event; emotional numbing and avoidance of reminders of that event; and physiological hyperarousal (APA, DSM-IV, 2000; WHO, ICD-10, 1991). Various studies have now established that PTSD can arise in children and adolescents following a wide range of traumatic events, including violent assaults, traffic accidents, shooting, serious illness, natural and man-made disasters, war, terrorist attacks, and physical or sexual abuse (see Perrin et al. 2000).

With its roots in studies of adult psychopathology, the diagnosis has been uneasily extended to apply to stress reactions in younger children. The major difficulty from the outset has been that some of the symptoms of PTSD are developmentally inappropriate for younger people. Indeed, the younger the child, the less appropriate the criteria. In this context, Scheeringa, and colleagues (1995, 2003) developed and evaluated an alternative set of criteria for diagnosing PTSD in very young children, based on parental report of observable behaviour.

Re-experiencing

Is seen as being manifested if one of the following is present: posttraumatic play; re-enactment of the trauma; recurrent recollection of the traumatic event; nightmares; flashbacks, and distress at exposure to reminders of the event.

Numbing

Is present if one of the following is manifested: constriction of play; socially more withdrawn; restricted range of affect; loss of previously acquired developmental skill.

Increased arousal

Is noted if one of the following is present: night terrors; difficulty getting off to sleep; night waking; decreased concentration; hypervigilance; exaggerated startle response.

A new subset of **new fears and aggression** was suggested and is said to be present if one of the following is recorded: new aggression; new separation anxiety; fear of toileting alone; fear of the dark, or any other unrelated new fear.

Carefully conducted studies from Scheeringa's group (Scheeringa et al. 1995, 2003), and others (Ohmi et al. 2002, Meiser-Stedman et al. 2008) suggest that these criteria are a sensitive, reliable, and valid means of diagnosing very young children's traumatic stress responses (Scheeringa 2008).

Incidence and prevalence of PTSD in children

Given that PTSD has only been recognized as occurring in young people since the late 1980s, there are not many studies to inform us as to how common it is. The *Jupiter* cruise ship sunk in Athens harbour on 21 October 1988 with 400 British school children on board. Just over half the surviving teenagers developed PTSD, mainly in the first few months. Many others were troubled by partial PTSD and had other disorders such as anxiety and depression (Yule et al. 2000). In other words, under certain circumstances, the incidence of PTSD can be high. It does also occur following accidents such as road traffic crashes, and the average rate of PTSD in six British studies is around 25-30% (Yule 2000). In many such road traffic accidents, children who survive may also be bereaved.

However, PTSD is relatively uncommon in the population as a whole. In the recent National Survey of 10,000 British children, the estimated prevalence rate was around 1% (Meltzer, Gatward, Goodman and Ford 2000).

Long term outcome

When PTSD was first described in adults, it was initially assumed that it would not be seen in children and young people (Garmezy and Rutter 1985). This was because up until that time hardly any clinical researchers had asked children directly about the largely inner distress they were experiencing. Instead, they had interviewed parents and teachers and, as we now know, children do not often confide their worries in adults who, in turn, grossly underestimate the levels of distress.

Thus, studies like those of the survivors of the *Jupiter* shipping disaster, by using well-standardised diagnostic techniques, clearly demonstrated that PTSD can be a significant consequence of a life-threatening experience. Moreover, the seven-year follow-up of the *Jupiter* survivors discovered that a significant minority of children (17%) still met strict criteria for a diagnosis of PTSD (Yule, Bolton et al. 2000).

For the purposes of the present chapter, the 33-year follow-up of the people who survived the coal tip disaster of Aberfan is even more relevant (Morgan et al. 2003). Coincidentally, also on the 21 October but in 1966, just as school was starting, the tip slid down the Welsh mountainside engulfing the school and killing 116 children and 28 adults. One hundred and forty-three primary school children survived, but scarcely a family in that tightly-knit community escaped the aftermath of the disaster. When re-examined 33 years later, 29% of the survivors contacted still had PTSD.

It looks as if a truly overwhelming and life threatening experience that actually involved heavy loss of life really can lead to long term problems in adjustment. For our purposes, we need to be aware that when a young person is involved in an accident or disaster that also involves loss of life of people known to the young person, then pathological grief reactions may occur.

Assessment

Careful diagnosis involving the use of standard procedures has been influential in getting the nature and extent of the traumatic stress reactions in children fully recognized. With proper assessment and diagnosis come better opportunities for effective treatment. When preparing to see a child for the first time, the clinician should try to get as much documentation as possible. That might include newspaper descriptions of what happened, television footage, architects plans, or eye-witness accounts. This helps focus the discussion on what happened. It is important to spend time separately with the child and the parents as often children try to protect their parents by underplaying their distress.

A standard family, personal and developmental history; an account of what happened in the incident; and an account of how the child is currently behaving are taken from the parents. This may include a standard interview schedule such as the PTSD component of the Anxiety and Depression Interview Schedule for Children (ADIS-C, Silverman and Albano 1996).

When children are seen alone, after spending a few minutes talking to them about themselves, their school, their friends, their likes and dislikes, they can be reminded that they have come to the clinic because of something scary that happened to them, and so after a very few minutes they are asked if they are ready and the clinician can say 'Now tell me about it'. It has been our experience over the years that when you show children respect and indicate that you are there to take them seriously, then they are amazing in being able to recall not only what happened, but also how they were feeling then and subsequently. At a suitable point, those children who are old enough to read independently can be asked to complete a few questionnaires on traumatic stress symptoms, anxiety, depression and traumatic grief. This helps in the diagnosis as well as providing a baseline against which response to treatment can be measured.

Sometimes, and especially with younger children, it can be helpful to ask them to draw a bit of what happened or to act it out with toys. One protocol that describes such an approach is that by Pynoos and Eth (1986). Note that one is not 'interpreting' what the child draws, but it can be easier for children to talk about what happened when they are drawing or acting it out with miniature people or other toys.

Child traumatic grief

Having noted that sudden, unexpected, violent deaths are often experienced as traumatic bereavement, there is also the issue of whether the subsequent grieving is different from ordinary bereavement. Some years ago (Prigerson et al. 1999) the concept of traumatic grief was suggested. It overlapped with depression and anxiety but differed from both. Above all, people experiencing traumatic grief showed considerable separation distress coupled with traumatic distress. They continued to yearn for the dead person and often their grieving seemed 'stuck'. They could not think about the dead person without memories of the traumatic death intruding and interfering with adjustment.

While professionals debate whether it is better to call this 'complicated grief' or 'traumatic grief', it became clear that children and young people also show similar reactions. Consideration of the needs of young people bereaved in the September 11, 2001 terrorist attacks in New York and Washington has accelerated the investigations of traumatic grief in children (Melham et al. 2007, Cohen et al. 2006, Brown et al. 2008 and Goodman and Brown 2008).

The emerging consensus is that following a traumatic bereavement, young people can sometimes also react with complicated and traumatic grief reactions. In addition to many of the symptoms of PTSD, depression and anxiety, they have preoccupying thoughts about the dead person, anger about the death, feelings that the dead person is still around, and all these interfere with normal grieving. The lack of consensus has meant that, until very recently, there has been no agreed way of measuring traumatic grief in children. However, there are now at least three measures under development – the Traumatic Grief Inventory for Children (Dyregrov et al. 2001; Dillen et al. 2009); the Inventory of Complicated Grief (Melham et al. 2007); and the Extended Grief Inventory (Layne et al. in press).

To date, the indications are that children are most at risk of developing traumatic grief: if they have suffered an earlier bereavement; the death was violent; the deceased was a close relative; the young person perceived that their own life had been threatened (Brown et al. 2008). The reaction overlaps with feelings of depression, anxiety and anger but is still different. It is related to the severity of the trauma as perceived by the child.

Crisis intervention

It would be good to think that early intervention can prevent the development of the worst traumatic stress reactions, but sadly there is insufficient evidence to be clear about this. Indeed, there has been quite a heated debate in the adult literature which suggests that some early interventions may stop normal healing processes taking place (Raphael and Wilson 2000). We should be clear that the literature, flawed and incomplete as it is, does not address traumatic grief or even children (Yule 2001).

Having acknowledged that, our view is that when a traumatic death occurs, there are things that can be done almost immediately, although not necessarily directly with the child. The child needs safety and security. They should have as many personal possessions available as possible. In particular, they should have access to photos of the dead parent. Where one parent has killed the other, clear decisions need to be taken about whether or not they should visit the perpetrator in prison – and if so, then never unsupervised. Arrangements should be made for them to attend the funeral and participate as appropriate to their age. Once settled, additional therapy should be considered. If of school age, then liaison with the teachers is vital to explain why the child may have problems concentrating, and why they may breakdown when something in a lesson reminds them of what happened. The child may need to be given an acceptable cover story to explain to others what happened.

If one is faced with a group of children who have witnessed the death of a school friend or teacher, then it makes sense to see the whole group together. An initial, structured meeting a few days after the death can be very helpful in clarifying for children what actually happened. It is characteristic of sudden traumatic events, that memory may be vivid but also patchy. Helping children share their memories as well as their reactions can place the event in a better context. It can also be reassuring to learn that others are experiencing similar reactions.

Note that the evidence for this preventing later problems is scanty. There should not simply be a one-off 'debriefing' meeting. Rather, a structured meeting should be the start of a planned surveillance and longer term set of interventions (Yule and Gold1993). A format for conducting such an initial meeting in a school is described in Dyregrov (2008a) and further suggestions for group leaders are in Dyregrov (2003).

Individual and group treatment

In clinical practice, it is more common to be asked to intervene several months (or even years) after the traumatic event – either on an individual or group basis. Two recent reviews have highlighted the growing evidence for cognitive behavioural therapy (CBT) for the treatment of childhood posttraumatic stress reactions (Feeny et al. 2004; Stallard 2006). The National Institute for Clinical Excellence (NICE, 2005) also recommends that trauma-focused cognitive behaviour therapy (TF-CBT) be used; and notes that a different approach, eye movement desensitization and reprocessing (EMDR), shows some promise.

Cognitive Behaviour Therapy (CBT)

Trauma-focused CBT is a short term intervention, typically lasting between 12 – 18 weekly sessions, and may be delivered individually (eg Cohen 2004) or in a group setting (Stein et all. 2003). Approaches vary and a variety of techniques may be used, but common elements include psycho-education about the nature of PTSD and its treatment, behavioural activation, imaginal exposure to the traumatic event, *in-vivo* exposure to traumatic reminders, relaxation training, cognitive restructuring, and work with parents. Excellent clinical outcomes are reported (Stallard 2006).

The most recent treatment developments have elaborated on the cognitive processing of the emotional reactions, informed by findings from experimental cognitive psychology of memory and emotions. Ehlers and Clark's (2000) cognitive model of PTSD in adults specifies a number of important factors that may maintain symptoms, including: the disjointed nature of the trauma memory; unhelpful appraisals about the traumatic event and its consequences; and unhelpful attempts at coping. There is now evidence that this model, suitably adapted, applies well to children of about eight years and older (Meiser-Stedman et al. 2007, Bryant et al. 2007). In Cognitive Therapy for PTSD (Smith et al. 2007), these maintaining factors are directly targeted, and the treatment therefore has five main goals: 1) trauma memories need to be elaborated and integrated into autobiographical memory; 2) misappraisals of the trauma and/ or of PTSD symptoms need to be modified; 3) dysfunctional coping strategies that prevent memory elaboration, exacerbate symptoms, or hinder a reassessment of problematic appraisals need to be changed; 4) maladaptive beliefs of the parents with respect to the traumatic event and its sequelae need to be identified and modified, and 5) parents need to be recruited as co-therapists. This is achieved using a variety of developmentally appropriate techniques, with a particular emphasis on identifying and modifying unhelpful appraisals. The new appraisals are integrated into the trauma memory in order to update it. In a preliminary trial (Smith et al. 2007), very positive results were reported, with 90% of those who received treatment showing substantial improvement and losing their diagnosis of PTSD after 10 weeks of treatment.

This evidence base for treatment (see Feeny et al. 2004; Stallard 2006 for reviews) is based on studies of children who had developed PTSD, but were not bereaved. There is far less evidence relating to traumatic bereavement.

Clinical impression and research suggest however that in cases of traumatic bereavement, the traumatic stress reaction needs to be treated first in order to allow grieving to proceed (Dyregrov 2008). This is the approach used by Cohen and her colleagues, who have adapted their manualized treatment for child PTSD to encompass traumatic grief. Their trauma focused cognitive behaviour therapy was extended to cover aspects of bereavement counselling. They give eight sessions of CBT targeting the traumatic stress reactions followed by four sessions focusing on the grief. To date, there have been two open trials of their approach which show considerable promise (Cohen et al. 2004, 2006). Layne et al. (2008) have described a related approach for working with war-exposed adolescents. The case study below illustrates a similar approach that we have found useful. More systematic studies are now needed.

Eye Movement Desensitization and Reprocessing (EMDR)

EMDR treatment was developed by Shapiro (1995) and its application to children has been described by Tinker and Wilson (1999) and Morris-Smith (2002). In this paradigm, a child is asked to imagine the worst moment in the traumatic event. Having got the scene firmly fixed in mind, the child then has to follow the therapist's fingers as they are rhythmically passed in front of the child's face. The child is instructed to let the images change in whatever way happens. In as far as there is any underlying rationale for this treatment, it appears to involve a mixture of exposure and distraction – or 'dual attention' as the manual prefers. While EMDR is endorsed by NICE (2005) for use with adults, to date there are no published accounts of randomized controlled trials with children and adolescents. As with all techniques that have no clear rationale, caution has to be exercised. However, if symptomatic relief can really be attained in a few brief sessions, then the approach needs to be carefully evaluated.

Michael – a case of traumatic bereavement

Twelve year old Michael was referred to the local Child and Adolescent Mental Health Service by his school, who were concerned that since transfer from primary school, he had not settled well, appeared isolated, and had been getting into trouble for fighting. He was occasionally tearful; at other times, he would lash out at others. School were aware of a recent family bereavement, but gave no further details. With mother's agreement, a referral requesting 'anger management and possible grief counselling' was made.

Assessment

Michael was very reserved during the initial joint meeting with his mother, and he asked that she speak to the clinician first. He completed some questionnaires while his mother was being interviewed.

Interviewed alone, mother said that her parents had died in a car crash some 18 months previously. They had picked Michael up from school to take him to football practice. Driving along a country road, they were hit head–on by an oncoming truck. Her mother died instantly; her father, who was driving, died in hospital the following day. Michael was sitting in the back of the car. He sustained serious cuts and bruising, but was otherwise unhurt. He was freed from the car by fire-crew, taken by ambulance to hospital, where he was met by his parents, and discharged home the same day. He did not want to go to his grandparents' funeral.

Prior to his grandparents' death, Michael had been a well-adjusted and happy boy. His parents had separated when Michael was two years old. Grandparents had lived nearby, and they had been supportive in the aftermath of the parents' separation, stepping in to provide childcare and practical support when needed. Michael had been especially close to his grandfather.

Michael's mother reported that after the crash, he appeared 'frightened of everything' – he was jumpy and restless. He appeared tired all the time, but wanted to delay going to bed. Mum heard him screaming during the night, but when she asked him about it, he told her that he could not remember. He was tearful at times, but he usually cried alone, in his bedroom. Mum had asked Michael if he wanted to go to the funeral, but he said no; and he had not visited the graves since then. She tried hard not to get upset in front of Michael because he would simply get up and leave the room. He refused to talk about the accident, or his granddad – becoming angry if the topic was raised. He could now travel by car, but had not been back to the site of the crash. He had given up his football. He was generally 'wound up and on edge', and was irritable with other children at school, and with his mum at home.

The initial assessment was helpful in clarifying that although Michael's mother was grieving the sudden death of both parents, she was not herself suffering from a post traumatic stress reaction. She was very concerned for Michael, whom she described as a 'changed character'.

Seen alone afterwards, Michael was far easier to engage than in the initial family meeting, and agreed that he had come to talk about the crash and his grandparents. He remembered the accident 'as if it was yesterday'. It took very little encouragement for him to say what had happened in the accident – he gave a fairly detailed account, becoming tearful as he did so.

He was congratulated on his bravery in telling what had happened. The clinician said that she wanted to hear more about Michael's grandparents, but first wanted to ask more questions about how Michael had been feeling and thinking over the last month. A structured interview was used to enquire about symptoms of PTSD. When asked directly, Michael said that that he had vivid and upsetting pictures of the crash pop into his mind nearly every day. He said that he used to 'hear' his granddad groaning. He had nightmares about once a week of the crash itself, and he usually woke up in a panic at the point where he had been trapped in the car. During the day, he tried to get rid of the pictures by thinking of other things. Sometimes, the images seemed to just pop into his mind out of the blue; at other times there were obvious triggers such as approaching the stretch of road where the crash happened, and photos of his grandparents. He tried to stay away from all sorts of triggers. Talking about what happened was too upsetting, so he refused to talk to his mother. Michael said that whenever he started to remember something nice about his grandparents, an image of them injured or dead in the car popped into mind. Consequently, he was avoiding all discussion or reminders of his grandparents – not just reminders of the crash. At school, he had been teased, and he agreed that he lost his temper sometimes. He said that teachers didn't understand, and he got the blame all the time.

Towards the end of the assessment, Michael was invited to talk about his grandparents, and he told of how granddad used to help out with football while granny cooked his favourite food. Nothing was the same now; he missed them, and felt sad, angry, and confused.

Formulation

Michael clearly met the diagnostic criteria for PTSD. He showed the three classic symptom clusters of intrusive memories (nightmares and daytime images), avoidance (trying not to talk about the crash, staying away from reminders), and arousal (increased irritability and poor concentration). These symptoms were causing disruption to peer and family relationships, and adversely affecting his academic attainment.

Since it appeared that Michael's traumatic memories were interfering with grieving, it was decided to prioritise these symptoms in treatment, followed by a grief-focused intervention as necessary.

Over the initial sessions, a number of factors that were maintaining Michael's PTSD – derived from the extended cognitive model described above – were identified. His memory of the crash was disjointed and patchy. He believed that his intrusive images were a sign that he must be going crazy. In later sessions, he described feeling very guilty about the crash, reasoning that it was his fault, because if his grandparents had not picked him up from school, then the crash would not have occurred. Michael's avoidance of trauma-related material was understandable, but the unintended effect was that he failed to 'update' the trauma memory, and so intrusive recollections persisted. Michael was very worried about his mother. They had been close prior to the crash, he recognized that she was upset, and he did not want to upset her further.

Trauma-focused intervention

Particular attention was paid at the beginning to normalizing Michael's reactions, and providing information about PTSD (including leaflets). Michael quickly came to realize that he was not going crazy. Michael was helped to understand that his avoidance of reminders was having the unintended effect of keeping his symptoms going – once he understood this, imaginal exposure and narrative techniques were used to help him 'get the memory out into the open' so that it could be updated. Particular attention was paid at this stage to his guilt feelings, using pie charts to identify all the factors involved in the crash. As he became more accustomed to talking about the crash in sessions, he was encouraged to discuss it with his mother. Towards the end of this phase of the treatment, Michael was helped to return to the scene of the crash, and he was able to contrast the differences between his memory of the scene and the current reality, and thus to update his trauma memory.

Grief-focused intervention

In the second phase of intervention, the focus shifted onto grief work. Michael was able to do this because his guilt had resolved and he was far less troubled by intrusive memories. He was encouraged to recall positive memories of both grandparents. This was helped by Michael bringing in some photos of them, some including him as a younger child. He had been left some treasured mementos such as granddad's football whistle: he brought some of these into a session. Discussion of granddad's role in the family revealed just how much Michael had loved football, and how much he was missing it now. He decided that his grandfather would have wanted him to continue playing, and decided to re-start by joining a junior Sunday league. Michael deeply regretted not having been to the funeral, as he felt that he had not had a chance to say goodbye. He was helped to write a letter to them in sessions. Now that Michael felt stronger, he told his mother that he wanted to go and see his grandparents' grave.

Witnessing father killing mother

A particular form of traumatic grief

Domestic violence remains a major source of distress and psychopathology in children. Within these tempestuous relationships, young children often witness the violence and may even be its target. Many young children, being the centres of their own developing worlds, blame themselves for what they see. Being small and powerless, they cannot intervene to protect their parents.

Harris-Hendriks, Black, and Kaplan (2000) have estimated that in England and Wales every year some 50 children are orphaned when one parent kills the other – most commonly the father killing the mother. As a result of their clinical expertise, they were able systematically to report on over 400 children and their study is a model of how good, careful clinical investigation can contribute substantially to our knowledge.

When the death is discovered, the alleged perpetrator is taken into custody. The house is sealed off as a scene of crime. Someone has to look after the child or children who may have been the only witnesses to what happened – but who is going to do so, even on a temporary basis? If the child is looked after by a paternal relative, they may try to revile the mother's character to justify what the father did; if a maternal relative takes over, the child hears how dreadful their father is. The child gets caught between two very emotional sets of relatives. Neither parent is there to comfort the child, let alone begin to explain anything. It can even be that the child has none of their favourite toys or comforters if they remain at the scene.

Moreover, as a potential witness, the police will want to take evidence from the child as soon as practicable. Even though the Crown Prosecution Services advice on 'Achieving Best Evidence' nowadays allows the interviews to be taped and, if necessary, presented as evidence-in-chief (so that the child does not have to appear in the court), it is still a potentially distressing experience.

At the same time, if it is decided that the child should be placed in the care of the local authority and usually with foster carers, the child is having to adapt to new carers who did not know the parents. Often, in our experience, such carers feel inhibited about helping the child talk about what happened. If the child has nightmares about blood, what should the carer say? If the child talks about the stabbing, should they ignore it or help the child clarify what happened? This is the sort of scenario that often presents to the Child Traumatic Stress Clinic.

The case of Harry illustrates some of the issues and shows how we respond to a crisis.

Case study – Harry

The clinic received an urgent request from a social worker who had been allocated Harry, a 3½ year old boy who had been found covered in blood sitting next to his dead mother. The father had been arrested and later charged with her murder. The killing had occurred less than 48 hours previously and the social worker asked whether we could provide therapy for Harry.

We immediately and clearly said, 'No'. That was not what the little boy most needed at this point in time. Until he was settled in a good permanent placement and the court case had been settled, there was little point in embarking on any formal 'therapy'. Rather, the therapist was very happy to consult with the foster carer as to how she was managing the little boy and to advise her on any concerns she had.

So it was that the therapist met with the foster carer and Harry on a few occasions over the next year. Not surprisingly, given the background of violence, Harry had been neglected and had not reached many of his appropriate social milestones. With firm, loving care, he quickly settled in the foster home. He was able to talk about his mum and a little about what he saw. He was reassured that what his dad did was not Harry's fault. The foster carer became attached to Harry and he to her, but she was due to retire and so Child Care proceedings were initiated, and Harry was freed for adoption. By then, he was much more settled and making good progress at nursery school.

At their request, the therapist met with the prospective adoptive parents and discussed with them some of the issues they may face in the future with Harry. He will need to revisit his understanding of what happened at various points throughout childhood and adolescence. It may be that various things unexpectedly trigger distressing reactions and recollections, and he may need help with managing these. Thus, they should enquire about the availability of Child and Adolescent Mental Health Services in their area so that should Harry get upset, some help is forthcoming quickly, bypassing any waiting list.

There are times when specialist 'therapy' is best placed in reserve so that normal healing processes can occur.

Concluding comments

The past twenty years have seen a dramatic change in the way children who have been traumatically bereaved can be helped (Dyregrov 2008a, 2008b). In the same way that our understanding of bereavement in childhood has improved – as seen in other chapters in this text – our understanding of traumatic stress reactions has developed rapidly. There is considerable agreement about what stress reactions are shown by children aged eight years and over. There is still a lot to learn about how they manifest in much younger children. With clearer diagnosis, we have learned that serious stress reactions can be quite common in children following particular traumatic incidents. Even though children can be very resilient, we must not assume that all are, as shown by the longitudinal studies mentioned earlier. For some children, the effects of a traumatic incident can last for many years.

Fortunately, along with the better ways of assessing stress reactions has come very powerful ways of treating them. Compared to less focused treatments of years ago, the new ways are grounded in good theory and evidence of outcome, and are generally fairly brief. Six to ten sessions is the usual length. Where bereavement is involved, this gets more complicated. This is particularly the case when the child loses one or both parents and has to be found a new permanent home. While helping the child to settle in, it may be necessary o postpone active intervention until that has been achieved.

This progress has come about because people have studied the presenting problems and the outcomes in detail. To do this, they had to develop appropriate, brief, but valid measures to capture the essence of the child's distress. Measures such as the Child Impact of Event Scale (see www.childrenandwar. org) made it possible to screen children who can read. Other self-completed measures of anxiety and depression were also very helpful. As yet, there are no similar measures of grief in children although we are currently developing an inventory of traumatic grief for children and adolescents. Tools to investigate traumatic stress and grief in younger children are urgently needed. As they become available, so will we be able to test out which are the best ways of helping children affected by traumatic bereavement.

References

American Psychiatric Association (1980) *Diagnostic and Statistical Manual of Mental Disorders* (3rd Edition). Washington, DC: APA.

American Psychiatric Association (1987) *Diagnostic and Statistical Manual of Mental Disorders* (3rd Edition - Revised). Washington, DC: APA.

Brown, E.J., Amaya-Jackson, L., Cohen, J. et al. (2008) Childhood traumatic grief: A multi-site empirical examination of the construct and its correlates. *Death Studies*, **32**: 899–923.

Brown, J. and Goodman, R.F. (2005) Childhood traumatic grief: An exploration of the construct in children bereaved on September 11. *Journal of Clinical Child and Adolescent Psychology*, **34**: 248–259.

Cohen, J.A., Mannarino, A.P. and Deblinger, E. (2006) *Treating Trauma and Traumatic Grief in Children and Adolescents*. New York: The Guilford Press.

Cohen, J.A., Mannarino, A.P. and Knudsen, K. (2004) Treating childhood traumatic grief. A pilot study. *Journal of the American Academy of Child and Adolescent Psychiatry*, **43**: 1225–1233.

Cohen, J.A., Mannarino, A.P. and Staron, V.R. (2006) A pilot study of Modified Cognitive-Behavioral Therapy for Childhood Traumatic Grief (CBT-CTG). *Journal of the American Academy of Child and Adolescent Psychiatry*, **45**: 1465–1473.

Dillen, L., Fontaine, L.J.R. and Verhofstadt-Deneve, L. (2009) Confirming the distinctiveness of complicated grief from depression and anxiety among adolescents. *Death Studies* (in press).

Dyregrov, A. (2003) *Psychological Debriefing: A Leader's Guide for Small Group Crisis Intervention*. Ellicott City, MD: Chevron.

Dyregrov, A. (2008a) *Grief in Children: A Handbook for Adults*. (2nd Edition) London: Jessica Kingsley Publishers.

Dyregrov, A. (2008b) *Grief in Young Children: A Handbook for Adults*. London: Jessica Kingsley Publishers.

Dyregrov, A., Yule, W., Smith, P., Perrin, S., Gjestad, R. and Prigerson, H. (2001) Traumatic Grief Inventory for Children (TGIC) Bergen: Children and War Foundation(cf www.childrenandwar.org).

Ehlers, A., and Clark, D.M. (2000) A cognitive model of posttraumatic stress disorder. *Behaviour Research and Therapy*, **38**: 319–345.

Feeny, N.C., Foa, E.B., Treadwell, K.R., and March, J. (2004) Posttraumatic Stress Disorder in Youth: A Critical Review of the Cognitive and Behavioral Treatment Outcome Literature. *Professional Psychology: Research and Practice*, **35**: 466–476.

Garmezy, N. and Rutter, M. (1985) Acute reactions to stress. In Rutter, M. and Hersov, L., (eds), *Child and Adolescent Psychiatry: Modern Approaches (2nd Edition)*. Oxford: Blackwell (pp. 152–176).

Goodman, R.F. and Brown, E.J. (2008) Service and science in times of crisis: Developing, planning and implementing a clinical research program for children traumatically bereaved after 9/11. *Death Studies*, **32**: 154–180.

Harris-Hendriks, J., Black, D. and Kaplan, T. (2000) *When Father Kills Mother* (2nd edition). London: Routledge.

Jones, J.C. and Barlow, D.H. (1992) A new model of Posttraumatic Stress Disorder. In Saigh P.A. (ed) *Posttraumatic Stress Disorder: A Behavioral Approach to Assessment and Treatment*, pp. 147–165. New York: Macmillan.

Layne, C.M., Savjak, N., Saltzman, W.R. and Pynoos, R.S. (2001) UCLA/BYU Extended Grief Inventory. University of California, Los Angeles. Available from Christopher. Layne@byu.edu.

Meiser-Stedman, R. (2002) Towards a cognitive-behavioral model of PTSD in children and adolescents. *Clinical Child and Family Psychology Review*, **5**: 217–232.

Meiser-Stedman, R., Smith, P., Glucksman, E., Yule, W. and Dalgleish, T. (2008) The Posttraumatic Stress Disorder Diagnosis in Preschool- and Elementary School-Age Children Exposed to Motor Vehicle Accidents. *American Journal of Psychiatry*, **165**: 1326–1337.

Melham, N.M., Moritz, G., Walker, M., Shear, M.K. and Brent, D. (2007) Phenomenology and correlates of complicated grief in children and adolescents. *Journal of the American Academy of Child and Adolescent Psychiatry*, **46**: 493–499.

Meltzer, H., Gatward, R., Goodman, R. and Ford, T. (2000) *Mental health of children and adolescents in Great Britain*. London: The Stationery Office.

Morgan, L., Scourfield, J., Williams, D., Jasper, A. and Lewis, G. (2003) The Aberfandisaster: 33-year follow-up of survivors. *British Journal of Psychiatry*, **182**: 532–536.

Morris-Smith, J. (ed) (2002) EMDR: Clinical applications with children. *Association for Child Psychology and Psychiatry*, Occasional Paper No. 19.

Prigerson, H.G., Shear, M.K., Jacobs, C.F. et al. (1999) Consensus criteria for traumatic grief. *British Journal of Psychiatry*, **174**: 67–73.

Ohmi, H., Kojima, S., Awai, Y. et al. (2002) A: Post-traumatic stress disorder in pre-school aged children after a gas explosion. *Eur J Pediatr*, **161**(12): 643–648.

Perrin, S., Smith, P., and Yule, W. (2000) Practitioner review: The assessment and treatment of post-traumatic stress disorder in children and adolescents. *Journal of Child Psychology and Psychiatry,* **41**: 277–289.

Pynoos, R.S., and Eth, S. (1986) Witness to violence: The child interview. *Journal of the American Academy of Child and Adolescent Psychiatry,* **25**: 306–319.

Raphael, B. and Wilson, J. (eds) (2000) *Psychological Debriefing: Theory Practice and Evidence.* Cambridge: Cambridge University Press.

Saigh, P.A. (1987a). In-vitro flooding of an adolescent's posttraumatic stress disorder. *Journal of Clinical Child Psychology,* **16**: 147–150.

Saigh, P.A. (1992) The behavioral treatment of child and adolescent posttraumatic stress disorder. *Advances in Behaviour Research and Therapy,* **14**: 247–275.

Saigh, P.A., Yule, W. and Inamdar, S.C. (1996) Imaginal flooding of traumatized children and adolescents. *Journal of School Psychology,* **34**: 163–183.

Scheeringa, M., Zeanah, C.H., Myers, L. and Putnam, F. (2003) New findings on alternative criteria for PTSD in preschool children. *Journal of the American Academy of Child and Adolescent Psychiatry,* **42**: 561–570.

Scheeringa, M.S. (2008) Developmental considerations for diagnosing PTSD and acute stress disorder in preschool and school-age children (Editorial) *American Journal of Psychiatry,* **165**: 1237–1239.

Scheeringa, M.S., Zeanah, C.H., Drell, M.J. and Larrieu, J.A. (1995) Two approaches to the diagnosis of postttraumatic stress disorder in infancy and early childhood. *Journal of the American Academy of Child and Adolescent Psychiatry,* **34**: 191–200.

Shapiro, F. (1995) *Eye Movement Desensitization and Reprocessing: Basic Principles, Protocols and Procedures.* New York: The Guilford Press.

Silverman, W.K. and Albano, A.M. (1996) Anxiety Disorder Interview Schedule for DSM-IV: Child and Parent Interview Schedule San Antonio, TX: *The Psychological Corporation.*

Smith, P., Dyregrov, A., Yule, W., Perrin, S., Gupta, L. and Gjestad, R. (1999) *A Manual for Teaching Survival Techniques to Child Survivors of Wars and Major Disasters.* Bergen, Norway: Foundation for Children and War.

Smith, P., Perrin, S. and Yule, W. (1999) Therapy Matters: Cognitive behaviour therapy for post traumatic stress disorder. *Child Psychology and Psychiatry Review,* **4**: 177–182.

Smith, P., Yule, W., Perrin, S., Tranah, T., Dalgleish, T. and Clark, D.M. (2007) Cognitive Behavior Therapy for PTSD in Children and Adolescents: A Randomized Controlled Trial. *J. Amer. Acad. Child Adol. Psychiat.,* **46**: 1051–1061.

Stallard, P. (2006). Psychological interventions for post traumatic stress reactions in children and young people: a review of randomised controlled trials. *Clinical Psychology Review,* **26**: 895–911.

Stein, B.D., Jaycox, L.H., Kataoka, S.H. et al. (2003) A mental health intervention for schoolchildren exposed to violence: a randomized controlled trial. *JAMA,* **290**: 603–611.

Tinker, R.H. and Wilson, S.A. (1999) *Through the Eyes of a Child: EMDR With Children.* New York: Norton.

World Health Organization (1991) International Classification of Diseases – 10th Edition. WHO: Geneva.

Yule, W. (2001) When disaster strikes – the need to be "wise before the event": Crisis intervention with children and adolescents. *Advances in Mind-Body Medicine,* **17** (3): 191–196.

Yule, W., Bolton, D., Udwin, O., Boyle, S., O'Ryan, D. and Nurrish, J.(2000) The long-term psychological effects of a disaster experienced in adolescence: I: The incidence and course of post traumatic stress disorder. *Journal of Child psychology and Psychiatry,* **41**: 503–511.

Yule, W. and Gold, A. (1993) *Wise Before the Event: Coping with Crises in Schools.* London: Calouste Gulbenkian Foundation.

Chapter 17

Helping the family following suicide

Kari Dyregrov and Atle Dyregrov

Even if someone had dropped an atom bomb in the middle of our community centre, we could not have been more affected...
(A father speaking one and a half years after losing his 14-year old son by suicide)

Individual effects of a suicide

The fact that a parent or sibling chooses to end his or her life is threatening and devastating to those left behind. Parkes (1998) emphasized that in the wake of a traumatic loss such as a suicide, there are possibilities that the grief process can go awry. The word 'trauma' itself indicates that an event is a shock. In addition there are several other circumstances and qualities associated with suicidal deaths that make them traumatic; they occur suddenly and unexpectedly, there is a perceived lack of control, the events are of out of the ordinary, and they create long-lasting problems. Thus it is important that the impact of this particular mode of death be understood and recognized, in order to respond adequately to those who need help, either on an individual or familial level.

Existential crisis

The brutal upheaval after traumatic losses may make great demands on bereaveds' capacity to confront and handle what has happened, cognitively as well as emotionally. Results from the Norwegian nationwide 'Support and Care Study' (Dyregrov and Dyregrov 2005; Dyregrov, Nordanger, and Dyregrov 2003), documented that one and a half year after the sudden death of an offspring/sibling by suicide (< 30 years), bereaved parents and siblings reported serious existential, psychological, physical, and social problems.

Post traumatic stress disorder

This nationwide study found that half of those bereaved by suicide suffered from levels of post-traumatic psychological distress indicating risk of PTSD (Dyregrov et al. 2003). Common post-traumatic reactions are; unwanted thoughts and images (intrusive reactions), strong anxiety (arousal reactions), as well as denial of the event and its consequences (avoidance reactions). Many also experienced psychic distress such as anxiety and insomnia, or severe depression. Sudden, untimely, preventable, and violent suicidal death may also lead to what is proposed as the syndrome of prolonged grief (Prigerson, Vanderwerker, and Maciejewski 2008). The bereaved are preoccupied with thoughts of the deceased, search and yearn for the person, experience disbelief about the death, are stunned by it, and have difficulties in accepting the death. In our study, 78% of the parents who lost their offspring to suicide scored above the cut-off level for risk of complicated grief at one and a half years following the loss (Dyregrov et al. 2003).

Physical illness

Increased muscular activity may explain why muscular-skeletal problems such as headaches and bodily pain are commonly experienced. Increased susceptibility to infectious diseases, cancer, or diseases of the cardiovascular system is seen after a suicide due to a suppression of the immune system. Another feature is an increase in sick leave from work and hospital admissions associated with increased physical illness, as well as an increased risk of early death (Li, Precht, Mortensen, and Olsen 2003). In the Support and Care Study, 62% of all parents scored above the cut-off score for high levels of psychosocial and physical complaints (Dyregrov et al. 2003).

Social difficulties

In addition, the bereaved often experience long-lasting social difficulties, for example with their social identity and social relations, as well as problems with social interaction in the family (Demi and Howell 1991). As reported in other studies, one of the main findings in the Support and Care Study was that bereaved individuals withdrew and isolated themselves from others (Dyregrov 2003; Dyregrov and Dyregrov 2008), both from people outside the family, and from one another inside the family. In addition, members of their social network withdrew from them. It seems that those bereaved by suicide become more isolated than other bereaved groups because of stigmatization or 'self-stigmatization', feelings of guilt, shame, anger, rejection, or loss of energy to socialize. Unfortunately, social and emotional withdrawal often acts as a barrier to accepting offers of social support and professional assistance.

The existential crisis that compels the bereaved to reorganize or change their cognitive 'schemas', may lead to a change of attitudes and values that result in changes being made to social life. Such processes may lead to the dismissal of relationships and friends and to less social life. Another explanation for a decline in social interaction may be isolation due to increased physical illness and changes in life events (Dyregrov et al. 2003; Dyregrov 2003).

Research has documented that child and adolescent development may be impeded by the lack of emotional accessibility of parents because of their grief and trauma reactions following suicide. Pfeffer and colleagues (1997) reported that, after a suicide in the family, between 25-40% of children and adolescents fulfil criteria for a diagnosis of PTSD. Also, children and adolescents may suddenly lose an important role model in a sibling or a parent in years of developmental importance. Thus, the suicide may trigger an identity crisis in the younger members of the family. Enduring guilt, anger and distress, and significant disturbances in self-esteem may increase the occurrence of depression and chronic illness. Children and adolescents who lose a close family member to suicide often drop out of school for a period, or experience academic difficulties. However, the individual reactions of children must always be viewed in a familial and parental context (Dyregrov and Dyregrov 2005).

Effects of suicide on the family

Communication difficulties

The level of communication in the family, and thus the prospects for mutual support within the family system, is closely related to parental attitudes towards the loss. In particular, difficulties between spouses, different grieving patterns, or feelings of guilt or reproach for the death will impact seriously on the family climate. Common difficulties among partners after the loss of a child by suicide are: fathers' concern and worry about the grief of mothers, the anger of mothers because the fathers do not share their grief, initial breakdowns in communication, loss of sexual intimacy, and general irritability between partners. Different grieving patterns often involve women employing strategies to confront the loss, whereas men often cope through more avoidant behaviour. Thus, women who wish to talk about and share their feelings about the death may criticize their male partners who instead prefer to work hard. Without knowledge of the most 'typical grieving patterns' of women and men, partners may criticize each other for not reacting appropriately to the loss, for dwelling upon the death, or for lack of understanding. Open communication and mutual support within the family seem to be imperative to the individual's and family's integrity following a suicide.

The question of why?

Family members will seek the answer to the question of why the suicide happened. Striving to find the answer, children and adults will often question the extent to which they, or the other surviving family members, contributed to the fatal outcome. Children may believe that their parent abandoned them because of something they did or said. Adolescents may feel intense anger, or blame the surviving parent because they did not do enough to help the parent or sibling who committed suicide. People bereaved by suicide often become obsessed with the 'if onlys' that could have brought about a different outcome. Thoughts that are devastating for the bereaved may seem completely irrational to outsiders. Families who are unable to ventilate or discuss these strong feelings and thoughts within the family need professional help to create a healthier climate for communication (Nelson and Frantz 1996).

Change of roles

After the initial shock and distress following the suicide, many caretakers are not able to resume their parenting role or day-to-day activities. This can mean that children's ability to mourn the death and express their feelings and reactions related to the loss is often severely restricted by their concerns for parental welfare. In fact, the demands on the parent(s) may be so great that the needs of surviving children can easily be forgotten or overlooked. Children may undertake the parental role for months, or even years.

Moreover, mutual support in the family may be impeded by parents' or children's catastrophic anxiety resulting in exaggerated attention or overprotective behaviour. Well-intended acts of parents, who want to protect their children from pain and sorrow, often worsen the family climate. In line with other studies (Rakic 1992, Sethi and Bhargava 2003), our study (Dyregrov and Dyregrov 2005) showed that bereaved children also seek to protect their grief-stricken caregivers, long after the suicide. In order not to stir painful memories and emotions in their parent/parents, children often restrain themselves from mentioning the death or the dead even though this conflicts with their desire to talk. If they express their need for parental support, they may feel guilty about making such demands.

Because the need to understand *why* seems to be a reaction specific to suicide, it is vital for the family functioning to create a shared acknowledgement of the reality of the death in the family (Dyregrov 2001). However, secrecy about the death or lack of open communication may result in interminable mourning and permit a 'ghost' to become an integral member of the family system. Children and adolescents may have knowledge of previous suicide attempts of siblings that the parents do not share, or the surviving parent may mourn an unresolved conflict that made the spouse kill him/herself. If 'forbidden knowledge' prevents a shared environment of communication and understanding about the suicide, this may nurture problems within the family.

The opportunity to express thoughts and feelings about a loss to others may contribute considerably to the healing of the biographical disruption caused by the event (Neimeyer 2000). How well the family manages to communicate about the loss and attend to individual family members will largely depend on the family's pre-existing coping and communication patterns. Research shows that the more expressive and sharing family members are, the closer they feel to one another in the wake of a suicide. Although couples that value open communication may show stronger grief reactions in the first phase after the loss than couples that do not, they seem to cope better over time. 'Disengaged' or 'conflicted' families experience greater distance while cohesive or expressive families report more closeness to one another following suicide. The greater the disengagement and level of conflict the younger members of the family perceive, the more distant they feel from their parents. Conversely, the more expressive and sharing family members are, the closer they feel to one another. Thus, if family members are able to act openly and share feelings and thoughts with one another, they may move through the grieving process within an accepting and supporting family atmosphere.

Difficulties, such as a tendency towards isolation and family interaction and communication problems following a suicide in the family, may necessitate professional assistance. However, it is important to know what kind of help and support the bereaved themselves perceive to be necessary after a suicide in the family.

What kind of help and support do families want?

The suicide bereaved in the Norwegian Support and Care Study expressed a strong need for both formal (professional) and informal (social network) assistance in dealing with their loss (Dyregrov 2002, 2003), as others also have found (McMenamy, Jordan, and Mitchell 2008; Provini, Everett, and Pfeffer 2000; Wilson and Clark 2005). When asked to describe ideal professional help, the bereaved highlighted the following aspects.

They wished for:

- immediate outreach help from trained personnel
- information about the event and reactions that may arise
- various kinds of assistance

- help for bereaved children
- the opportunity to meet with others who have experienced the same or a similar situation
- help over time.

Immediate and outreach help

The bereaved want early community outreach help without having to take the first initiative. They claim that they are not able to ask for the help that they really need, even if helpers tell them to 'contact us if you need help'. Several important reasons may explain why the bereaved do not seek help to the degree that they deem necessary. First, exhaustion and loss of energy make many bereaved people incapable of initiating contact with community services. Thus, paradoxically, one of the reasons why they need help becomes a barrier to obtaining it. A second reason why suicide bereaved want to be contacted and offered help is probably due to the pervading stigma of suicide. Internalizations of shame and guilt, and possible prejudice shown by others may account for their reluctance to seek the help they need. Also, they may not know what kind of professional help they need, or what is available. Well aware of their changing needs for help during the bereavement process, the parents and siblings in our study emphasized that assistance should be repeatedly offered during the first year.

Information

Immediately after the suicide, bereaved relatives often feel in desperate need of different kinds of information. They ask for information on medical aspects of the death, the process of mourning, and possible side effects of the death on family members and family systems. In particular, they ask for advice concerning help for children and difficulties between spouses following suicide in the family. Bereaved families want both verbal and written information.

Various kinds of assistance

The bereaved families in our study clearly confirmed that the focus of help had not been adequately tailored to all their concerns. Besides psycho-educative information, the parents asked for help with existential, practical, economic, and legal matters, as well as therapeutic interventions and advice. In order to reduce distress, nightmares, flashbacks etc., more specific psychological help and advice was desired by the parents. This included a wish for 'psychological help' for themselves, their children, and for the family as a whole.

Help for bereaved children

The parents in the Support and Care Study asked for different kinds of advice on how to help and deal with surviving siblings. Two thirds of the parents wanted more help for their children, and 45% wanted psychological help, emphasizing the necessity of focusing more on this vulnerable group. Parents also wanted family counselling to increase harmony and resolve conflicts in the parent-child relationship, and to get support for coping with the needs of their child. Bereaved adolescents requested support as separate individuals, and help in avoiding the taking on of parental roles and responsibilities for younger siblings.

Opportunities to meet with others

Many bereaved want to meet with others who have experienced the same or a similar situation. The bereaved families in our study requested help to mobilize social networks or establish contact with grief groups, or organizations for the bereaved. They asked that local authorities should take steps to organize links between those bereaved by suicide, either one to one, or in support groups. They emphasized the importance of learning from the unique experiences of other bereaved people concerning 'how to survive the pain'.

Help over time

The duration of follow-up is a central issue, and most of the bereaved claim that an ideal follow-up would need to encompass a lengthy time perspective. The questionnaire data in our study showed that 73% wished they had been offered contact with authorities and, if necessary, help from professionals for at least one year. In the interviews, a high proportion also pleaded for support and help over 'at 'least two years', or 'as long as it is needed', or 'the rest of our lives'. The reality is that the bereaved are often supported during the first weeks while they are in shock or busy with the funeral etc. only to be left alone to face the harsh reality after the first month. Most of the network support also stops after a few months.

In summary, the bereaved had the following advice for health care professionals about how they could help (see Box 17.1).

Box 17.1 Advice from those bereaved by suicide to health and social care professionals

- Be organized – develop or instigate routines for response
- Be proactive, don't wait for us to come to you
- Don't swamp us with help initially and then leave us with nothing
- Be there when the reality of the death sets in
- Be flexible – listen to what we need
- Provide us with information (What will happen? Where and from whom will we get help? What are 'normal' grief reactions – individual, family, gender differences?)
- Help our children and help us to help them
- Do not forget the extended family
- Help us get in contact with others who have experienced the same bereavement
- Be available to us for at least a year.

Immediate help for children

If children are present at the scene when a dead person is found, it is important to limit their exposure to the event, though not by force. They should be led away from the scene, have an adult they trust with them, and have what happened explained to them in concrete terms adjusted to their age and maturity. Do not use phrases such as: 'It will be all right' or 'It could have been worse'. Providing them with information about what will happen in the hours and days to come will be appropriate for school children, while younger children need the presence of an adult to balance the anxiety that witnessing powerful adult reactions to the death can invoke in them. If no one from the family can be with them, a neighbour, adult friend, or other adult they trust (e.g. a teacher) should stay with them until a family member can come.

In the immediate situation, the child will need reassurance that adults they know will be there for them, and that they will not die, or take their life as the suicide victim did. It is extremely important to create a caring, safe environment for the child where they can get the support they want, where they can have a lap to sit on and close physical comfort to counterbalance the increased arousal created by the sudden death. They should not, however, be given false assurances or any hope of the person returning or being alive.

Telling a child about a suicide

If the child was not present when the suicide happened or when the body was found, it is important not to postpone telling them what has happened. Although it may be hard to tell them openly and directly about what happened, this is often harder on the adults who face this task than for the children being told.

Depending on the age and maturity of the child, one has to choose what words to use, what context to place the suicide in, and how much detail one relates. The child does not need to have all the details, but does need to know that the death was caused by the deceased themselves, and how it was done. There is no reason to go into detail unless being asked directly by the child. If they do ask and it is too difficult to answer, one response could be 'I do not know exactly how to explain this to you. I will think about this and then tell you later today or tomorrow'. This allows time to think and, if possible, to consult with someone else who knows the child or who has more experience of such situations. If there is a suicide letter, it will be important to tell the child about this, even if there is something written that they will not understand until they are older. This should be explained to the child.

It is important to convey that the adults did not do this because of lack of love for the children, but because things felt so bad for them that not even the thought of the children could keep them from taking their own life. There are various strategies for how to choose to explain a suicide and the strategy must to some extent be based on the circumstances of the actual death. When there is a history of depression, we use a metaphor where a person's thoughts are likened to leaves in autumn that wither and die (Dyregrov 2008b).

Whatever explanation is used, it is important to allow the child to ask questions, and to return to the subject within the first few days to check out what the child has understood. Children may harbour a conviction that their own thoughts or behaviour somehow contributed to the death so it is important to tell them that nothing they have done, said, or thought, or not done, said, or thought led to what happened.

Case study

When Julia was 12- years old her mother committed suicide after a long history of being manic-depressive. Her mother used to wave from the window as Julia left for school in the morning but on the morning of the suicide, she did not come to the window. Julia blamed herself for not having understood that there was something wrong that morning and felt that perhaps if she had returned instead of going to school it would not have happened. She also blamed herself for being 'moody', thus contributing to her mother being sad. Because no one noticed or knew how she blamed herself, it was not until she entered therapy that her self-blame could be addressed through cognitive techniques. She was then able to say: 'Mother was sad from before I was born'. If during the immediate follow-up, she had received more reassurance that nothing she did, or did not do, had anything to do with the suicide, her self-blame might have been prevented.

Including children in rituals

Participation in rituals makes the loss real, has great symbolic significance, and provides an opportunity for expression of thoughts and feelings that were provoked by the suddenness of the death. Elsewhere we have written in more detail about how and when to include children in rituals (Dyregrov 1996). We wish to emphasize the importance of including children whenever possible. A child that is only six months of age will not have a conscious experience nor have a memory of being in present in the viewing of a father that committed suicide. However, 15 years later that child is 15 ½ and it may be very important to learn that 'yes, you were present in the room when we said farewell'.

Viewing the body

Where an adult can view a dead body there is no reason to exclude a child. It is, however, important to prepare children properly for the experience. This preparation should include being prepared for sensory impressions (what the room will be like, in what ways the dead person looks different from usual, how the person will feel cold if touched, etc.), how adults or the children themselves may react, and what they can bring to put in the coffin (drawing, letter, other memento). They should also have adult support during the ritual. It may be helpful for someone other than the parent to be present. Following the ritual, children must have a chance to express their reactions and to receive answers to their questions e.g. 'what happens to the body now?'

Talking with children

It is often wise to use open questions in conversations with children, or to ask them to tell you what you have explained to them, or to tell you what they have understood about what happened. This can reveal misperceptions and misunderstandings that can be corrected. Initially, it will be important to help the child and other family members to get a 'grip' on what has happened. It may be important to gather and record information which may be significant and hard for the child to find later on. A child has less understanding of the chronology of events and may need special help from adults to organize what happened along a 'time line'. A child will revaluate what happened and their own involvement

Box 17.2 Adults need to understand

- ◆ how children react to death
- ◆ how important it is that children get honest information about what has happened and what will happen in the near future
- ◆ what children understand at different stages of their development
- ◆ how they cope with grief
- ◆ that children may:
  - need to sleep in their parent's bedroom for a time
  - become more clingy for a period
  - behave as if nothing has happened
  - and will need stability in daily routines.

in what happened as they grow older, and have a fuller understanding of the long-term consequences of the event.

Information for adults

To help children cope with what happened it is important that the parents, the surviving parent or other caretaker receive adequate assistance to help them care for their children.

It may be difficult for an adult overwhelmed by what has happened to talk with children about what is most painful. From our clinical work we know that children often refrain from talking about their loss because they sense that their parents or remaining parent easily become upset or that it causes them pain. For this reason it is important that other adults are there for them if they want to talk about their longing or pain related to the loss (see Box 17.2).

Early help

Following the immediate phase one should be careful about forcing an emotional processing of the event on the child. Let children do this at their own pace, but be aware of their signals and check with them whether they are harbouring fantasies or are experiencing intrusive images or thoughts about what happened. Children's capacity to regulate their emotions develops gradually, and they often avoid long conversations about something that is painful. If they do not want to talk there may be several reasons for this, for example, it is too painful, they do not feel the need, they are afraid of not being understood, they feel guilty. Be patient, do not pressure them to talk but be ready to follow up on their cues. If the child seems to be doing well in school and does not start to isolate him/herself and the child's behaviour does not undergo serious changes, there are usually no reasons for concern.

Sometimes the family's reactions to a death by suicide may necessitate meetings with professionals or volunteers to facilitate or restore family communication. Provide the family with advice on how to access bereavement services and encourage them to talk to their family doctor. Early therapeutic help may help in preventing unnecessary long-term problems, and newer methods developed for complicated grief and posttraumatic stress problems may benefit children. Although resources are scarce, it is important to try to refer children sooner rather than later. In all therapy, it will be important to restore children's experience of control and predictability in their life (see Box 17.3).

Box 17.3 'First aid tips'

- Go through what happened to make sure that the child (and family) have an overview and understanding
- Follow up on thoughts the children experienced when they learned about what happened and afterwards
- If the children have taken in strong sensory impressions or have created strong fantasies based on what happened, e.g. observing a father shoot himself, let them express these in words or drawings. Provide them with simple self-help strategies to take control of these (see Stallard 2002)
- Ask about the reactions the children experienced when they learnt about what happened and afterwards. Sensitively describe normal reactions in order for children to be able to recognize these if they experience them. Be sure to say that children do not have to experience this to be normal, but that these reactions are what other children who have lost someone close have described
- Stimulate expression of thoughts and emotions through play, art activities, and rituals, and help the children develop a 'narrative' or story about what they have experienced
- If new facts about the death become known, inform the child
- Give the child suggestions about what others have done that has helped them, including talking with friends, advice about sleep, etc.
- Advise adult caregivers on how they can create stability in children's lives and how to make contact for further help
- Encourage contact with friends and help children think about how to explain what has happened to them.

In addition to the psycho-educative and supportive efforts aimed at the individual child, it is very important that the child bereaved by suicide is included in family communication about the suicide. Through open, honest, and direct communication about facts, and feelings about what happened, the children will be able to integrate the suicide as they go through the developmental phases in childhood and adolescence. It is important that children are given age-related support and help, and that the principles for help are applied at home, at school, or in the nursery. Further information on advice concerning bereaved children can be found in Dyregrov (2008a, b).

Help for the family bereaved by suicide

Work to help the family starts on the day of the suicide. The main aim is to ensure that family members are carefully looked after, and to start normalizing the situation in cooperation with the bereaved family. By reducing distress, and re-establishing a kind of order and structure, the individual and the family can be helped to restore function and 'a normal life'. It is very important that helpers map the aspects of the actual situation and encourage the individual and the family's strength and coping resources.

Emotional 'first aid' may be given at a hospital, by the ambulance personnel, the clergyman, crisis teams, or by local community health support workers. The bereaved should be met with calmness, support and empathy in a situation that is chaotic and unreal. Psychoeducative information should be provided for the bereaved from the day of the suicide, and repeated over time. To be able to comprehend and start re-constructing a world that has fallen apart, information about the death is essential. It is important to help family members access information to order and structure what happened.

Within a couple of days after the suicide, it may be appropriate to provide the family with more information. Initial advice and written information for the family are of utmost importance in contributing to the initiation of the grief process and to normalizing and possibly reducing traumatic reactions. It is important that guidance is provided early in order for parents to make decisions about whether children should see the deceased. Advice about when belongings of the deceased should be removed should also be provided early on, before well meaning friends and relatives start clearing things away too fast. Information about the importance of participation in rituals and the importance of including children in these should be provided. It is also important to give information about the inquest, post mortem, and other legal events that will take place during the first days following the death. It is important, in a sensitive manner, to prepare the bereaved for the existential crisis that many will experience with its ensuing trauma-, crisis-, and grief reactions. Later on, gender differences, problems related to family dynamics, children's reactions, and the way grief changes over time, should be stressed. However, professionals should not present these aspects in such a manner that people may feel there is something wrong with them if they do not encounter such problems. The timing, as well as the quantity and the quality of the information, must be attuned to the needs of the individual or family.

Ideally, every family bereaved by suicide should be offered the opportunity to meet with a grief counsellor to discuss family communication, the children's reactions and behaviour, and family dynamics. The frequency of the meetings should be adjusted to the needs of the individual family, but aim at contact close to memorial days (dates of birth and death) and major holidays. Counselling may include individual advice on the necessity of returning to painful places or activities, and discussion of common reactions connected to the birthday and death-day of the deceased. It is important to advise parents how to care for bereaved children, as well as to support and encourage their successful efforts. The bereaved need information about available psychosocial health care provision and how they may apply for additional help.

Prepare the family for situations and circumstances that they will encounter as time goes on (e.g. gender differences in grief, reactions of others, etc.). Because of the frequent disturbance of memory function in the wake of a traumatic loss, it is helpful to provide information both orally and in written form.

Helping agencies need to acknowledge that some families lack or have very restricted or unhelpful social networks, so that effort may be required to mobilize these. Professionals and volunteers can prepare the bereaved family for other people's often disappointing or hurtful reactions, and give advice on how to manage this. Finally, information about, and offers to attend support groups or NGO-support organisations may be provided through distribution of leaflets. Information about support groups such as 'Survivors of Bereavement by Suicide' (UK) can be very useful.

Conclusion

A suicide in the family is a devastating experience for the adults and children left behind, often resulting in a tremendous and long-lasting impact. As well as the individual suffering of family members, the family's communication and structure is also tested. Bereaved people ask for help from both professionals and social networks. They want immediate and outreach help from trained personnel, they seek information, various kinds of assistance, more help for children, the opportunity to meet with others who have been bereaved, and help provided over time. In order to secure adequate help for all families bereaved by suicide, routine community intervention programmes should be implemented.

Although we have outlined a philosophy of caring and a strategy for help, we wish to stress that every family is unique. Every individual and every family should be met and helped on the basis of their needs. The challenge for social network members and professionals alike is to withhold our own concepts about what families are experiencing and what help we think they need, and listen carefully to what they tell us.

References

Demi, A.S. and Howell, C. (1991) Hiding and healing: Resolving the suicide of a parent or sibling. *Archives of Psychiatric Nursing,* 5(6): 350–356.

Dyregrov, A. (2008a) *Grief in Young Children. A Handbook for Adults.* London: Jessica Kingsley Publishers.

Dyregrov, A. (2008b) *Grief in Children. A Handbook for Adults.* 2nd edition. London: Jessica Kingsley Publishers.

Dyregrov, A. (1996) Children's participation in rituals. *Bereavement Care,* 15: 2–5.

Dyregrov, A. (2001) Telling the truth or hiding the facts. An evaluation of current strategies for assisting children following adverse events. *Association for Child Psychology and Psychiatry Occasional papers, no. 17*: 25–38.

Dyregrov, K. (2002) Assistance from local authorities versus survivors' needs for support after suicide. *Death Studies,* 26: 647–669.

Dyregrov, K. and Dyregrov, A. (2005) Siblings after suicide – "the forgotten bereaved". *Suicide and Life Threatening Behaviour,* 35(6): 714–724.

Dyregrov, K. and Dyregrov, A. (2008) *Effective Grief and Bereavement Support: The Role of Family, Friends, Colleagues, Schools and Support Professionals.* London: Jessica Kingsley Publishers.

Dyregrov, K., Nordanger, D., and Dyregrov, A. (2003) Predictors of psychosocial distress after suicide, SIDS, and accidents. *Death studies,* 27: 143–165.

Li, J., Precht, D.H., Mortensen, P.B., and Olsen, J. (2003) Mortality in parents after death of a child in Denmark: a nationwide follow-up study. *The Lancet, 361,* **9355**: 363–367.

McMenamy, J.M., Jordan, J.R., and Mitchell, A.M. (2008) What do suicide survivors tell us they need? Results of a pilot study. *Suicide Life Threat Behavior,* 38(4): 375–389.

Neimeyer, R.A. (2000) Searching for the meaning of meaning: Grief therapy and the process of reconstruction. *Death Studies,* 24: 541–558.

Parkes, C.M. (1998) Coping with loss: Bereavement in adult life. *British Medical Journal,* 316: 856–859.

Pfeffer, C.R., Martins, P., Mann, J. et al. (1997) Child Survivors of Suicide: Psychosocial Characteristics. *Journal of American Academy of Child and Adolescent Psychiatry,* 36(1): 65–74.

Prigerson, H.G., Vanderwerker, L.C., and Maciejewski, P.K. (2008) A Case for Inclusion of Prolonged Grief Disorder in DSM-V. In Stroebe, M.S., Hansson, R.O., Schut, H. and

Stroebe, W. (eds), *Handbook of Bereavement Research and Practice*, pp. 165–186. Washington, DC: American Psychological Association.

Provini, C., Everett, J.R., and Pfeffer, C.R. (2000) Adults mourning suicide: Self-reported concerns about bereavement, needs for assistance, and help-seeking behavior. *Death Studies*, **24**: 1–9.

Rakic, A.S. (1992) *Sibling Survivors of Adolescent Suicide*. Dissertation Doctor of Philosophy, The California School of Professional Psychology Berkeley/Alameda.

Sethi, S. and Bhargava, S.C. (2003) Child and adolescent survivors of suicide. *Crisis*, **24**(1): 4–6.

Stallard, P. (2002) *Think good – feel good. A Cognitive Behaviour Therapy Workbook for Children and Young People*. West Sussex: John Wiley & Sons Ltd.

Survivors of Bereavement by Suicide (UK) www.UK-sobs.org.uk 0870 241 3337.

Wilson, A. and Clark, S. (2005) *South Australian Suicide Postvention Project. Report to Mental Health Services*. Report. Department of Health. Department of General Practice. University of Adelaide.

Chapter 18

Family liaison: when once has to be enough

Julie Ellison

What is family liaison?

Another day and another shocking headline; a murder, a rape, or a road death and another family's grief is played out in the newspapers. Once more police family liaison officers (FLO) are said to be comforting the family.

But who are these family liaison officers, and what do they do?

Family Liaison has always been a core policing function although for many years it was generally confined to homicide investigations. A police officer was assigned to liaise with the bereaved family and keep them updated of developments in the investigation. Most families want to know how the investigation into the death of their loved one is progressing. For some the grieving process cannot begin until the offender is brought to justice.

The primary role of FLOs is that of investigators. They must be able to elicit information from a shocked and traumatized family in an empathic and compassionate way.

In a murder investigation where time is of the essence and initial leads limited, information from friends and family may prove vital. Police officers refer to background information such as routines, hobbies, and habits as 'victimology' and it can be highly significant – if you can find out how the victims lived you may find out how they died.

Historically officers asked to perform this task received no training, and there were no guidelines to explain what was required of them. Although feedback from families was frequently good, some did not regard the service as satisfactory and the now infamous murder of Stephen Lawrence, an 18-year old black student stabbed in a racial gang attack in 1993, highlighted the deficiencies of the role.

The subsequent Public Inquiry (Macpherson 1999) made over 70 recommendations; many focusing on family liaison. The Metropolitan Police developed a comprehensive training programme to address these recommendations, and engaged the expertise of the St Christopher's Candle Project to deliver the bereavement input. Over 2,500 FLOs have attended the week-long courses, which started in 2000. The design of the course has been adapted and used for police forces in other parts of the UK and Eire.

A video entitled 'The Message' (Met. Police 2003), featuring bereaved families discussing their response to the death notification and the impact of the police investigation, is central to the training.

Family liaison officers continue to provide investigative expertise and support to families. Their role has developed further following disasters involving multiple fatalities such as 9/11, Bali, the Tsunami, and the 7/7 London Bombings, which have seen FLOs deployed nationally and internationally to families primarily to obtain identification evidence so that the remains of their loved one can be returned to them.

Nearly all bereaved families regard the notification of death as the most traumatic moment of their lives. Many Police Forces choose a FLO to break the bad news to a family, although it is not feasible to ensure a trained officer is always on duty. Sensitive news needs to be delivered as soon as possible, but it is vital to establish key details before speaking to a family, who usually want to know everything about the incident.

A dilemma arises over whether to delay notification until sufficient information is gathered, or risk the family being informed by another source, potentially with even less information than the Police. This is particularly pertinent if the media is present. Even without precise information, the Police are always the preferred option. They are able to contain the situation and have received some training in delivering bad news.

There is no easy way to deliver a death message, particularly if the death was sudden and traumatic. Frequently families are shocked and unable to comprehend the news which may have to be repeated several times. Adding to their distress, delays in viewing the body and funeral arrangements are common in criminal investigations, as forensic evidence needs to be collected. If the death was violent or involved a severe traumatic impact, the body may be disfigured. All these things can be difficult to explain to a family especially when children are present.

The following extract is taken from *Breaking Bad News (a Practical Guide for Delivering Death Messages to Families)*.

Prior to delivering the death message, the following points need to be considered:

- ◆ Establish that the right message is delivered to the right person
- ◆ Gather as much information about the circumstances of the incident to tell the family, including when/where the family can view the body
- ◆ Do not assume that neighbours are the best people to help the family or be with them when giving the message

◆ Religious or community leaders may be able to provide valuable cultural information and support

◆ Consider if communication issues need to be addressed by interpreters

◆ None of the above should delay delivery of the message if there is a chance of the family finding out from any other source.

(Metropolitan Police 2003)

Delivering bad news when children are present

When a police officer attends an address to deliver a death message, invariably their knowledge of the deceased and the incident is basic, but their knowledge of the next-of-kin may be even more basic, consisting of little more than a name. They may have no idea of who is at the address. For many adults the arrival of a police officer at the door will induce fear and inevitably herald bad news. But a child may react very differently. Their natural curiosity will be aroused, especially if the officer is in uniform. The officer faces the predicament of going ahead with the message or asking the child to leave the room. Too often, children are the forgotten victims. We know they are there, but how do we begin to explain to them the death of someone very special? Adults are often so bewildered and shocked themselves they are unable to help their children.

The FLOs training will have helped them prepare for such situations in advance. The family will probably look to them for advice; some may even ask the FLO to tell the child on their behalf. In these circumstances, the FLO will try to empower them to do this themselves. The police officer will only be a transitory presence in the child's life whereas the surviving parent will be there in the long days ahead. It will be of no use to the child if the only person able to address their questions is the police officer who is no longer there. The officer needs to recognize that the parent is asking for help and reassurance, and given time and support will tell their child.

Sometimes once has to be enough

The following case examples illustrate what can be achieved by FLOs even with limited contact with a family.

Case example 1

Mr and Mrs N lived in a flat with their four young sons; the youngest, 8 month old Jamie. When Mr N left early for work one morning, the children joined their mother dozing in bed following a late night feed with Jamie.

Mrs N woke to find the duvet and the bed on fire. She took hold of the older children and dragged them outside. She tried to return to Jamie, asleep in his cot, but was beaten back by flames and had to be restrained by neighbours. The Fire Brigade rescued Jamie but he died in hospital soon afterwards.

Family Liaison Officers were involved from the outset; providing support to the family at the hospital and helping medical staff break the news of Jamie's death to relatives arriving at the hospital. Early investigations suggested the duvet had been set on fire with a cigarette lighter. The parents confirmed their sons had a fascination with flames and had been known to play with matches.

Despite their own grief, they were anxious to avoid any sense of guilt or blame being attached to their sons, and to do everything they could to ease their pain. The FLOs discussed the possibility of the boys seeing their brother. Whilst not averse to the idea the parents had concerns about how their children would react to seeing Jamie, particularly as he had facial burns.

The boys were asked to bring a toy for their brother. The FLOs spoke to them first with their parents. They told them Jamie's body had stopped working. He was not asleep although it might look like he was. His body would not work any more, he had been too little to cope with the hot fire and had died. He was unable to speak or play with them and he would feel cold. His hands and face would have red marks from the fire.

Accompanied by the FLOs, the parents led their children into the room and lifted them up to see their brother. They gave him their toys and were allowed to touch and kiss him.

It was an emotional yet pivotal moment in the investigation, as one of the boys told Jamie he was sorry for starting the fire. Hugged by his parents they told him he was not to blame although they were sorry Jamie had died. The children were video interviewed for the Coroner's Inquest and were subsequently referred to the Traumatic Stress Clinic at the Maudsley Hospital. They attended Jamie's funeral and placed pictures they had drawn for him into his tiny coffin.

Case example 2

A traffic officer had to tell a woman her husband had died in a motorcycle collision on his way to work. She was at home alone when he delivered the news and was understandably distressed. Suddenly realizing her six-year old son was due home from school, she felt unable to break the news herself and asked the officer to do so on her behalf.

He reassured her that she would not be left alone, but gently questioned whether her son should hear such important news from a stranger rather than his mother.

With the officer's support the mother told the child herself. He remained with her until other relatives arrived, returning the next day to answer any further questions from mother and child. He agreed to retrieve an undamaged mirror from the motorbike as the child specifically requested something to remember his father by.

Conclusion

FLOs are not counsellors. If specialist support is required, FLOs can make arrangements for families to be put in touch with local agencies quickly and confidentially.

There are distinct limitations in what can be achieved when the intervention is brief, but experience has shown that the value of those interventions should not be underestimated. For families bereaved by sudden death, the police officer is a source of stability and reassurance. What they do, however short term, can make a very real difference.

References

Breaking Bad News (A Practical Guide for Delivering Death Messages to Families) (2003) London: A Metropolitan Police Service Publication.

Macpherson, W. (1999) The Stephen Lawrence Inquiry. London: HMSO.

The Message (2003) London: A Metropolitan Police Service Publication

Chapter 19.1

Sibling carer story

Julia Manning

The following is a personal account of a young woman's experiences following her mother's death when she became a carer to her younger siblings. This young woman has been supported by the Candle Project after she phoned us directly asking for help and advice. Both she and her younger siblings have taken part in individual counselling sessions and groups offered by the project and the support is ongoing.

The names of the individuals have been changed. Diane, who is in her late 20's, is the sibling carer of her two sisters, Jade 13 years old and May 11 years old.

'I am the eldest of nine children and I took legal responsibility for my two youngest sisters in August, 2003. Our mother died in April, 2003. Since then it has been up and down. I have no children of my own, I work full time and I am trying to cope with everyday life, plus make sure that my two sisters are cared for, they are 13 and 11 years old. The eldest, Jade, seems to have been caught in her grief for her mother, never talking about it yet it seems to be affecting her at school, at home, and just about all through her life generally. May is younger and due to move from primary to secondary school soon and I am worried about her, she talks a little more about our mother, but I don't know if they are okay, how do I know if they are doing okay, or if I'm doing it right?'

This was Diane's first contact with the project. She had phoned feeling desperate and wanting help, but she admitted it was a hard call to make. She did not want us to think she was unable to cope and that her sisters were at risk, but said she needed someone to hear how hard it was to be parenting her sisters, to be working full time, and that the worry of it all was becoming almost too much for her.

Diane revealed she had reached a point where she was questioning if she could provide the right care and support for her sisters. Could she meet their changing needs as they were growing up, and also meet her own? The Candle Project offered several sessions to Diane and to Jade and May to address these and other issues that had arisen since the death of their mother.

Diane's mother, Deborah, had nine children in all and largely brought them up as a single parent. For the most part the fathers have not been actively involved in their children's lives. Diane, the eldest, recalls her mother suffering from long-term emotional issues, which at times made Diane worry about her. Deborah was a vulnerable woman who had little support, who had started her family as a very young woman. Depression was a constant theme in her life. Over the years this became debilitating and she would show symptoms of anxiety. She had little support from extended family or partners so continued to raise her family on her own. Despite her illness, Diane recalls Deborah as a warm, loving mother who tried her best for her children.

Jade and May were the two youngest children and lived at home with their mother while older siblings moved away and became independent. Their childhood was at times difficult due to their mother's health issues and economic deprivation. They moved home frequently, at times staying in supported housing or hostels, or with family. As a result home life was often unsettled, with disruption to routines, schooling, and family contact. Deborah's mental and physical health was not good, and sometimes the statutory social care services would become involved through concerns for the children.

Diane and the girls describe how their mother's death has become a painful memory for them all;

> At home one day in April 2003, when Jade and May were eight and six-years old, their mother began to complain of chest pains and said she was finding it hard to breathe. She took herself out of the room and the girls thought she had gone to lie down, but some time later May found her mother slumped in the bathroom not moving. Both girls tried to help their mother but didn't quite know what to do. After calling a neighbour, an ambulance was also called, and their mother was taken to hospital where she died the same day. The girls can recall this day well, they remember mum being ill, and the image of her unable to move still haunts them both. She was too heavy for them to move and they were so young they felt frightened by what they found. It is also a worry and concern for Diane and causes her real upset when she pictures what her sisters must have experienced; she feels their pain and wishes it had never happened. It is still a day that all of them find hard to retell.

Diane remembers the immediate time after the death as busy and confusing. It wasn't clear who would sort her mother's belongings out, or who would care for Jade and May. The other siblings in the family were in their late teens or 20's and decided for themselves where they would live or with whom, but for Jade and May it was an unknown. It also felt chaotic as everyone in the family had their own opinion and ideas of how things should be arranged. Diane says that being the eldest she immediately felt a sense of responsibility for her youngest sisters, and perhaps a duty to her mother also, but weeks and months of uncertainty passed when the girls moved around between relatives before any permanent home was found.

Diane took the decision to apply for legal guardianship for Jade and May with the hope that eventually the three of them would live together. She also hoped this would settle any disagreements amongst family members as to where the girls should go, and avoid the two girls being taken into Social Services care, as this might have resulted in them being separated.

As Diane tells the story, she recalls how social workers again became involved after Deborah died, but Diane did not feel supported or guided through the legal process of becoming a guardian for her sisters. She now recognizes that it would have been beneficial for her to have had some guidance with this, but she feels that, perhaps because Social Services saw the children as in a safe and appropriate home with her, they withdrew their involvement quite soon.

Diane had left home many years previously; she had studied hard at her chosen career and had secured herself a skilled job, which was demanding but enjoyable. Living independently in a one bedroom flat she was making her own choices and was in control of her own future, something she now recognizes that she perhaps took for granted, and she can also see was a lifestyle her mother never achieved. The choices and decisions she faced after her mother's death were unexpected and at times difficult, and this was a lonely and confusing time for Diane.

Diane was granted Guardianship for Jade and May and they spent the first few years living in Diane's small flat. Diane then applied to her local authority to be re-housed, which involved extensive negotiations and many forms to fill in. They were finally given appropriate housing in 2006; they continue to live permanently together. Diane sees this as a major achievement.

Diane shares her mother's Christian faith, and feels this has been a central force in her determination and will to care for her sisters. However she continues to struggle with and question the new role she has taken on.

> '... Do I parent my sisters, or behave like a big sister? What is my role? Why should they listen to me about what they can or can't do or have, what time to be home, or who they can hang out with, or how much homework I think they should do? It is hard and causes lots of arguments and tension. But I worry about them so much, I just want them to be okay, to be happy'.

Diane feels that the constant pull between sisterly love and parental responsibility is an ongoing dialogue for her. In the life she has chosen, she will always be an older sister, and her determination to raise Jade and May well is paramount.

From the moment Diane became a sibling carer, she felt she had to juggle so many roles; the immediate financial, legal and housing issues that had to be resolved, the worries around holding down a full time job while running a home for three people, and the biggest, and perhaps most constant, worry of suddenly becoming solely responsible for a six and eight-year old. With this came the massive responsibility of meeting all their personal and emotional needs, especially around their grief for their mother, and finding ways to address the girls' feelings and future changes.

Diane found becoming a 'parent' was not an easy thing to do. She had no previous experience and no one to turn to for help, but she did quickly learn that the things children benefit from are routine, clear boundaries, and lots of love. The three of them found a way to work together, routines were established, and Jade and May learnt to trust Diane as their main carer and the person they could turn to. The school the girls attended was very supportive and helpful and they began to find shape and comfort in their new family structure. Older siblings would offer support and would have the girls to stay from time to time to give Diane a break.

Jade and May are now growing up, bringing new challenges for Diane. The transition from primary to secondary school for both girls was difficult and Diane needed to learn how to work with the education department. Supporting the now adolescent Jade and May is very different from supporting and cuddling six and eight-year olds. Diane finds disciplining the girls now they are teenagers causes a lot of tension and arguments. It has been at these times of change that Diane has felt insecure about her role and worried about getting it wrong.

Diane now attends the Sibling Carers Group at the Candle Project, (see Chapter 7), which provides a forum for carers in her position to share ideas and experiences and find support from others in a similar situation.

> 'Being their carer means I have to tell them what to do, but it doesn't mean they will listen to me. I have to make decisions about school or friends or going out and it is hard to know how to make the decision. My friends don't have teenage kids so there is no one to talk to that understands. The Candle group has been great for meeting other carers like me. I know my sisters won't necessarily thank me or understand my reasons for certain decisions I make, but I just want them to be safe, and I want to try and do this job well'.

Diane has had to change direction in her life. She is highly committed to her role as a carer, but can see her own personal life is not what she expected. Her faith and the extended family are important sources of support, but relationships are not easy and friends need to be understanding. She spoke about this recently at the group;

> 'Sometimes I wonder if we will sink or swim when things get really bad. Then I realise it will be okay, we'll just paddle along and get through it, and it will pass, until the next thing'.

Mountains and medals: a young person's journey

Emma Lupton with Durone Stokes

Durone Stokes is fourteen years old. He identifies as Black Caribbean British and lives in South East London with his mum, dad, and older sister and brother. Durone's eldest brother Aaron was murdered three years ago at the age of 24.

Durone came to the Candle Project for individual counselling before Aaron's funeral, which was delayed whilst a post-mortem was performed. Since that time Durone has regularly attended the Young People's Group; the following account is Durone's story, shared with the hope of helping professionals as well as other young people who may be going through similar experiences.

Waking up on the day after New Year's Day and hearing lots of people in the house, some screaming and crying, Durone knew that something was not right. He remembers his dad coming into the bedroom, climbing onto his father's lap and being told by him that he would not see his brother again. At first Durone did not know what this meant and remembers feeling shock and blocking out his dad's words when he said, 'Aaron is dead, he got stabbed'. Going downstairs, people were crying and apologizing as if it was their fault, and nothing made sense as usually family get-togethers were times when people would be smiling and having fun. Now every time there is a celebration it does not seem the same without Aaron. Durone imagines his brother getting older like the friends of Aaron's that the family still see.

Aaron no longer lived at home, but Durone was used to seeing his big brother nearly every other day. He remembers his visits; Aaron brought treats from the shop where he worked, and they played on the computer together. Remembering Aaron helps Durone, it feels good to know that he had 'a brother as great as him' and he enjoys wearing one of Aaron's jackets as 'it feels like he's hugging me'. Aaron was stabbed on New Year's Day in the hostel room where he had lived for nearly four years. Little information or details are known about what happened that evening, and nobody has been arrested to date for Aaron's murder.

One of the most difficult aspects of Durone's story is the difficulty of establishing a grief narrative because of the circumstances of this bereavement by murder:

> 'so the story is open, if you get what I mean, because there's no certainty to what happened, I don't know any certain facts, all I know is that my brother died, he was stabbed in the heart. If it was my way, justice would be Aaron not dying but the justice we need right now is for there to be a solution – it would be great if they could find and punish the person who did this to us. It's not that I want any punishment on anybody, it's just really hard on my family and me knowing that someone killed my brother and they're still out there and I don't know what they're doing. It's just really horrible and it really makes me angry'.

Durone speaks about how any death is hard but how 'when someone's life is taken away by someone else it is really harsh on a family'. Losing his brother by murder heightens his feelings of confusion and anger and the 'rollercoaster' of grief. Indeed the painful injustice of Aaron's death is amplified by the uncertainty and the constant struggle with not knowing what happened and the anguishing, unanswerable question of why:

> 'Every time I break down or cry I just say " why?" as if I'm expecting an answer but it's never going to be there'.

When Aaron died, Durone had just finished his first term of secondary school – a difficult transition stage for most young people. Returning after the holidays, it was hard being surrounded by teachers and peers who did not know him very well at such a difficult time. Carrying on with his normal routine was problematic; he knew that his mum said it would help to go to school and he did not want to make her feel bad, but he felt there was something guilt provoking and disrespectful to Aaron that life could go on.

Durone passed a dance exam with distinction shortly after Aaron's death and recognizes that Aaron inspired him. Durone feels rightly proud of his achievement and identifies that working for his exam was a way of channelling his emotions into activity. There were times when Durone did not want to get out of bed, or go to school, or do anything, he just wanted his brother back. Grief is messy and cannot be timetabled and so it is that even now some days are better than others:

> 'I want to be happy and I try to be a positive person but when you think of things it just knocks you down and it's really like a mountain to climb back up to your positive side. It just comes into my mind and I'm not feeling good, it's just horrible 'cos at school I thought I wouldn't have to worry about or think about what's happening at home, but it's just hard to work when that's on your mind. The funeral time was really weird and horrible as well cos my mind was in different places y'know, when I went back to school I'd think about how he looked at the funeral'.

Durone feels well supported at school by teachers and friends but powerful images and strong feelings such as weakness, anger, guilt and sadness can make it hard to concentrate. This was particularly so in the early days and around the time of the funeral. The post-mortem meant that the funeral took place about two months after Aaron's death. Durone had a counselling session at the Candle Project on the day he went with his family to view Aaron's body at the funeral directors. The worker prepared him that Aaron would not look the same, how he 'would be there physically but not there spiritually' and that he may seem paler. Thinking about his brother's body being cut open and seeing his swollen face and changed features was shocking but because of the counselling session, he felt able to take it in properly. Viewing Aaron's body: 'it didn't look like him and he wasn't there' and the funeral were both very painful but helpful markers on Durone's 'mountain climb'. Both helped him to accept the finality of Aaron's death:

> 'I used to think that no, he's still here, he's gotta be – maybe they've got the wrong person, it's not my brother that died – they say he's died but he's just gone on holiday for a really long time'.

After Aaron's funeral, Durone continued going to the Candle Project for individual counselling where 'you say everything you feel':

> 'it helps so much to be able to talk to someone that isn't going through what you're going through because you know that they're not going to feel upset with you saying it. You're letting feelings out of you and it was hard to control my emotions, so counselling helped with this'.

Durone finds talking with his mum and family most helpful, but the opportunity of talking to a stranger offered something different, especially in the early days after Aaron's death when as a family it was hard to talk. Durone is aware that as the youngest child, his parents shielded him from things and also how he wanted to protect his family from his upset because it hurt to see them cry. Counselling helped to open up new family conversations, often in the car coming home. He recalls surprise at finding out new details about Aaron's death and as he grows older he is renegotiating his story as part of the grieving process:

> 'When I look back three years ago when my brother died, we somehow didn't talk about him, and I think we've come a long way. Before we wouldn't say his name, it would be 'he' and now we use his name – it shows how strong we're getting as a family. It feels good, it feels like we're progressing and that strengthens me. I feel more confident and like I've achieved something out of this horrible time and when I say achieved, I don't mean in a gold medal way but in a sort of progressive way'.

Yet talking to Durone, a wholly impressive young person, there is definitely something of the gold medal quality to him. At times Durone almost seems surprised about how at the age of eleven he coped with his bereavement and 'puberty on top' and then sagely recognizes that as a fourteen-year old, going through this is still hard and unfair. It is clear that Durone's grief has taken him on a journey and although he recognizes that his 'enormous pain' will never go away, he has come to accept it and seems to be growing stronger around it:

> 'there's definitely no words to describe how big or how hurtful it is, it's just an enormous pain and I don't think it's going to go away, the pain doesn't heal but you get stronger as a person and then the pain is not as strong on you. Grief does make me stronger as a person, whenever there's a challenge I'll persevere because I know there's a greater pain and it does inspire me to work harder in my dancing, singing, and different things'.

Durone's experiences give him a perspective and insight that at times sets him apart from his peers; the everyday challenges that young people face and cause his friends to worry do not hold the same significance. This difference can make it hard to feel that friends really understand what's going on and sometimes their concern makes things feel worse when Durone wants to feel like everyone else. Durone currently attends the Young People's Group at the Candle Project, which provides a space where his experiences are normalized and he can gain support from other young people without feeling different:

> 'Candle always helped – every time I came away feeling better because there's so many kids around you that have gone through similar things, they may not have lost the same person but they're young and they've gone through having lost someone in their family and so you've already got a connection. It wasn't as hard to talk to them, I didn't feel weird because I'd lost my brother and I didn't feel like I had to hold back on what I was going to say 'cos they'd lost their person, someone close to them and I realised that I wasn't going to make them upset. It helps a lot knowing that even though you've got a counsellor, you've still got someone around your age that you're able to talk to. You can still be friends y'know, we're still normal and it's not like we're isolating ourselves from the world but it helps that we have that connection and we're able to talk to each other knowing that you actually understand from a kid's point of view and that's incredible'.

Durone's bereavement and experiences at the Young People's Group have led him to want to share with others how he has felt and help other people in the future, possibly through his music and dance.

> 'If I was to get a message across, I think that as long as young people trust people like their counsellors and have hope, then they will progress really well and things will get better. I'm still 14 and young and don't know everything, but from what I do know, I believe that with hope and trust in what you've got, your counsellors and your family, then I think you'll be alright'.

Chapter 20

Crossing the great barrier grief

Stewart Sinclair

Introduction and history

When my wife Susan died in 1994 of breast cancer at St Christopher's Hospice, my two children were four and seven years old. Our family had received much help from the hospice through her illness and beyond. It soon became apparent that there was a very significant gap in service provision for those who are parents of young and teenage children and have lost partners. Angela Paul and I were asked by the Candle Project to help establish a parent/carers group which started in 1999. Angela was a young African Caribbean mother of St. Lucian descent with two young children at the time of her husband Sean's death from skin cancer. Like my own family, they had received much assistance from St Christopher's, and Angela had also noticed the same gap in service for the bereaved parent, at a time when a deluge of sympathy, empathy, and offers are poured onto our children.

Important components of the practical structure, such as child care and transport

Much practical guidance can be found in the leaflet produced by the Child Bereavement Network, 'Setting up a facilitated self-help group' (2006). When bereavement overwhelms a family sometimes the daily practicalities of life fragment along different fault lines. If you do not have a motor car and you do not have easy access to professional or extended family child care help, when you are suddenly on your own, with a child or children, many things that were taken for granted as part of a shared relationship are shattered. Even at the bus or train station, how do you go to the toilet when you have a child or children and baggage? You no longer have a partner to help with the pushchair on the bus or coach, and you have to rely on a public who may or may not be inclined to assist. Of course single parents are familiar with these situations, but those who find themselves in this predicament through the death of a partner are not, and the psychological disablement can at times be enduring and profound and can generate unexpected stress and sadness and despair, perhaps when you are tired and waiting for a train that is endlessly delayed, and the bags are heavy, and the children are crying, and it is cold and raining.

With the help of volunteers who had been trained, selected, and Criminal Records Bureau checked, we were in a position to provide safe and reliable transport for those who needed it to attend each meeting; and at the meeting of the group itself all the children could be looked after by the volunteers. The 'looking after' is not just 'minding', it is actively involving the children in various stimulating games and crafts, and it encompasses an age range from baby to teenager.

The 'fall-out' is different for all of us, but the universal theme that emerged in planning and setting up the group was the crucial need to have time and space away from our children, but in the knowledge and comfort that they were nearby, in an environment with safe and secure child-care. Sometimes the atmosphere in the group can be grim, sometimes it is funny, and sometimes it just cannot be captured in words, but the eloquence of unwritten and sometimes unspoken sadness forms a strange alchemy that can only be found in a self-help group.

Key structural features of the group are:

+ Transport resources and a place to meet
+ Childcare services
+ Time and space away from our children
+ Feeling safe
+ Being comfortable if you are not articulate and being comfortable if you are
+ Feeling comfortable, whatever your background/gender
+ Helping to ease the sadness of isolation post-bereavement
+ Helping to assess the natural context of sadness and depression by using the group to help and monitor ourselves in a safe and informal environment.
+ Using group leaders, who if possible balance gender and ethnicity.

Operating a subtle and gentle hierarchy within a user control/self-help philosophy

We were not 'elected' as group facilitators, and we do not serve a set term of office. To counterbalance any tendency to autocracy, or over-controlling attitudes, there is a supervisory and accountability framework. The group facilitators report to and are supervised by a Candle Project worker. The Parent/Carer Group is an informal but structured partnership with the Candle Project.

In summary:

- A structure of management, however loose, needs to be formulated. For example, how many children will attend in order to confirm number of volunteers required
- The existence of a hierarchy is likely to be an important attribute for a parent/carer group. It is a lonely and desolate time and most of those who have joined our group have stated clearly that at least initially having semi-formal 'leaders' was a great comfort
- A clear route for referrals needs to be prepared, with some kind of filtration system to protect new and 'raw' members
- A rolling record is helpful to know who attended. It is the practice in our group to take notes of each meeting so that some continuity is preserved for big and little issues, as things easily get lost between meetings
- The core paradigm of the group is self-help, not user control.

Some individual anonymized 'grief histories'

Ralph

Ralph is a forty-six-year old African-Caribbean man whose family originate in St Kitts. He has three children, two boys and a girl, and his wife died of leukaemia. He works locally in the fast food industry and has struggled to keep his job, his house, and his car. He has not received much help from the extended family and he heard about the group through St Christopher's Hospice. On joining, he explained the struggles he had been having with almost every aspect of his life, but most of all described the loneliness of his daily existence. He said that the others in the group had helped ease the terrible burdens of this isolation and made him feel less 'alone', especially as he was now in contact with those who understood his predicament, without him having to say anything.

Since becoming a regular attender, Ralph has told all of us how he had found being soothed just by empathy was often enough to 're-charge his batteries' – so sometimes he would merely sit quietly and listen to others who were struggling with their loss. At other times he might actively contribute, but he has said that for him the group had been a vital component in the complex machinery that allows most of us to recover from tragedy. Ralph acknowledged that he had found it very difficult as a bereaved man to seek out help, and he had been amazed about how quickly he felt safe and comfortable.

Rebecca

Rebecca, a white woman in her thirties, was never married to her partner, but they had been living together for a very long time and had a twelve-year old son. She works in a local library. Her partner had committed suicide when there were no indications that anything was wrong. She described the utter desolation she had felt after the tragedy, of being overwhelmed by her own guilt that she had not detected any signs that might have alerted her to her partner's hidden turmoil and given her an opportunity to prevent him taking his own life.

Attempting to manage her own turbulent thoughts had been difficult enough, but she described in the group the almost impossibly sad task of trying to deal with her son's feelings when she herself was barely able to function. Rebecca said of the group that it was, 'the only place I have been able to come that deals with parents on a self-help basis …….. that is what I need. I am just not used to dealing with things on my own and that is why I come to the group'. She said the group had helped her keep her difficulties with her son in perspective, realizing that the repercussions of losing a parent had certain universal features in young children, whatever the cause of the death. She added that the gaps between the meetings, for her, allowed a 'yardstick' to measure her own recovery and adjustment, and to discuss with others how each person found their own pathway to this same process.

Sandra

Sandra has three children and her husband had died suddenly of an illness that was never fully understood. She joined the group because she wanted to be among those who were experiencing similar difficulties. She is a white middle class woman from a professional background who unexpectedly found her two boys 'going off the rails' as she described it. She said she had come from a high-achieving, comfortable environment and devastating as her and her family's loss was, she thought she could deal with it all. She openly told the group how wrong she was, and how her two adolescent boys had become difficult and challenging after their father's death. She said in one group meeting, 'never in my wildest dreams did I think I would be fishing any of my children out of a police station at two am in the morning because they had been caught vandalizing property at a railway station'.

Being able to talk about this in the group had been an immense help to her, and had caused her to reconsider her own vulnerabilities and needs in relation to herself, as well as her family. She said the group absolved her of feelings of guilt about having failed her children, and made her realize she was not a 'superwoman' and that her children needed help and so did she. She said for her the group was a catalyst for change and a very positive experience.

Boundary setting, assimilation, and direction

How does the group recruit and assimilate new members who may be at different points of adjustment post-bereavement?

The group provides a quiet and safe time, away from children, where issues and feelings can be discussed openly in a confidential and supportive atmosphere amongst people who are united by personal tragedy.

The main aim of the group is to try and offer a forum and space for developing a self-support framework, where everything can be discussed without feeling stupid or silly.

Sensitivity to the different stages that people are at is vital, and we are learning as we grow to tackle the variety of things that those attending bring to the meetings. We are also learning the processes for the group as new people join, as others leave, and some drop in and drop out and drop in again. The 'funnelling' process of assessment and referral is undertaken by the professional Candle team.

Each session begins with introductions. Even if we all know each other. we can forget in the gaps between meetings, and if new people have joined we give them time to talk about their circumstances, and how long ago it was that their partner died. However, some have not wanted to do this immediately. It is important to recognize that we all have different vulnerabilities. A particularly raw area is when relatively newly bereaved people join the group, and listen to others talk about wanting or having new relationships, or perhaps confessing that actually they had an awful relationship with their deceased partner – considerable sensitivity is required in such circumstances. In the group we try to regularly mention this feature of bereavement.

Inevitably, a 'core' group has formed from those who nearly always appear for meetings, but we have been as aware as we can to not allow an informal hierarchy to emerge within the group between the regulars and the not so regulars. Most of the assimilation process is social common sense. The following points may be of guidance to others:

- Our experience suggests that it is important to have a professional referral and assessment process
- A system of supervision also allows a process of evaluation and monitoring to occur. We do not want accidentally to do more harm than good, nor is it safe to assume that because it is self-help, it is automatically good

- It is important to have a process of introduction at each session to help all involved know where they, and others, are on the bereavement spectrum

- Be aware of cultural, religious, and class issues

- Be aware of gender issues in setting up a group and in attracting referrals and assimilating new people. The gender imbalance in professional bereavement services is startling, and it is important not to replicate this process in a self-help setting

- A mechanism for following up new referrals who do not continue is very helpful in developing a group.

How participants' common needs and different needs determine the length of individual attendance at the group

Within our own histories of grief, we all have unique experiences of tragedy and reconstruction, and the self-help group has given us all a forum to express our individual grief paradigm and to seek equally individual succour from our involvement. For many of us, struggling to raise our children on our own, being part of the group has become a continuum where we compare notes and disasters about our children, our in-laws, about Christmas, and about holidays, and about love and loss. Some attenders have found new relationships but remained in the group, others have not. Others, with older children, have left when these children have passed into adulthood. A number of people drop in and out of the group, one man said he felt that it was really helpful to him to know the group was there and he could just turn up if he felt like it at a particular time. He said he had found no other source of support that could offer this and did not make him feel guilty if he just did not feel like turning up at a particular session. He added that it was also comfortable to be in a group where there are other men.

Rules including potential child protection issues and mental health issues

Although informal the following guidelines have been agreed for the group. The main points are available in a leaflet that is sent to those referred.

- All those involved are told that if there are significant child protection or mental health concerns, we will bring this to the attention of the professional team

- No discrimination

- Respect for others; everyone to have their own time to talk

- To try to be on time
- All information excepting the issue in the first bullet point is confidential
- Friends cannot attend.

Handing over the group to new facilitators

After a number of years of facilitating the group, both Angela and I felt it was time to think about handing over our roles to new facilitators. This was no easy task because for us and the group members, it was another stage in the adjustment process of bereavement. Also it was the challenge of finding suitable new people, and handing over the 'baby' knowing it will be nurtured quite differently by these 'new' facilitators. However, that is the nature of self-help groups, and it is an inherently healthy process, and 'baby' is, we understand, doing fine.

Topic agenda

Examples of topics that regularly emerge in sessions:

- Practical issues such as state benefits, and the lack of them
- The political agenda around single parenthood
- The deficits of the education and health services
- Children growing up and their sexuality
- Adjusting to grief and loss
- Having feelings about possible new relationships
- How do we know if our children are being naughty or just normal?
- Struggles with loneliness and sadness.

Summary

Usually ten to sixteen people attend each session, and we meet about six times per year; three of these meetings have child-care support. The logistics of organizing these supported sessions is formidable involving volunteer drivers, volunteer child care workers, and administrative help with post, and so on. Other gatherings during the year are more informal; picnics, a visit to a theme park, and a Christmas party. Generally we have maintained a very diverse ethnic, class, and gender mix.

Notes are taken at each formal session to keep a loose continuity, but they also serve as a semi-formal method for us to begin to evaluate how we ourselves are functioning, and to see if things regularly arise that are not being addressed.

Because bad luck and tragedy do not discriminate, amongst those who attend we are bound to have one or two people who present challenges through personality problems or other difficulties that may have little association with their bereavement, or perhaps their bereavement exacerbates these underlying problems. Usually the group process can contain such situations, but any group should have a strategy for containing individuals who may not respect conventional boundaries. The security of the professional framework serves many purposes including providing support in such situations and a conduit to other services.

An abridged and revised version from the first edition. Dedicated to the memory of Susan Dennison and Sean Paul.

Reference

Kraus, F., Sinclair, S. (2006) 'Setting up a facilitated self-help group'. London: Childhood Bereavement Network.

Index